Patterns of Rogerian Knowing

Edited by

Mary Madrid

National League for Nursing Press • New York
Pub. No. 15-6886

To the living presence of Martha E. Rogers.

The views expressed in this publication represent the
views of the authors and do not necessarily reflect the
official views of the National League for Nursing.

Library of Congress Cataloging-in-Publication Data

Patterns of Rogerian knowing / edited by Mary Madrid.
     p.   cm.
  "Pub. no. 15-6886."
  Includes bibliographical references and index.
  ISBN 0-88737-688-6
  1. Nursing—Philosophy. 2. Rogers, Martha E. 3. Holistic
nursing. I. Madrid, Mary.
  RT84.5.P395   1997
  610.73'01—dc21   96-29676
                                                              CIP

This book was set in 10 point Garamond Book by Publications Development
Company of Texas. The designer was Allan Graubard. The printer was
Bookcrafters. The cover was designed by Lauren Stevens.

Printed in the United States of America

Contributors List

Marcia Andersen, RN, PhD, CS, FAAN
President
Personalized Nursing Corporation, P.C.
Ann Arbor, Michigan

Elizabeth Ann Manhart Barrett, RN, PhD,
    FAAN
Professor and Coordinator
Center for Nursing Research
Hunter Bellevue School of Nursing
Hunter College of the City University of
    New York
New York, New York

Kaye Bultemeier, PhD, RNCS
Family Nurse Practitioner
Women's Health Associates
Oak Ridge, Tennessee

Howard K. Butcher, RN, PhD, CS
Assistant Professor
School of Nursing
Pacific Lutheran University
Tacoma, Washington

Judith Treschuk Carboni, RN, MSN, CS
Doctoral Candidate
University of Rhode Island
Kingston, Rhode Island

Cynthia Caroselli, RN, PhD
Assistant Professor
Coordinator of Graduate Nursing
    Administration
Division of Nursing
New York University
New York, New York

W. Richard Cowling III, RN, PhD
Associate Dean for Graduate Programs
School of Nursing
Virginia Commonwealth University
Richmond, Virginia

Jacqueline Fawcett, RN, PhD, FAAN
Professor
University of Pennsylvania
School of Nursing
Philadelphia, Pennsylvania

Steven Field, MD
Clinical Assistant Professor of Medicine
New York University School of Medicine
Attending Physician, Tisch Hospital/NYU
    Medical Center
Attending Physician, Bellevue Hospital
New York, New York

Jeanie Gold, RN, MSN, HNC
Adjunct Professor of Nursing
School of Nursing
Bergen Community College
Paramus, New Jersey

Jeffrey L. Gold, MD, FACP
Clinical Assistant Professor
University of Medicine and Dentistry
New Jersey Medical School
Newark, New Jersey
Clinical Assistant Professor
Seton Hall University
School of Graduate Medical Education
South Orange, New Jersey
Private Practice, Internal Medicine
Clifton, New Jersey

Joanne Griffin, RN, PhD
Associate Professor
Division of Nursing
School of Education
New York University
New York, New York

Sarah Gueldner, RN, DSN, FAAN
Professor and Director of the School
    of Nursing
The Pennsylvania State University
University Park, Pennsylvania

Effie S. Hanchett, RN, PhD
Associate Professor
College of Nursing
Wayne State University
Detroit, Michigan

Marie Hastings-Tolsma, RN, PhD
Associate Professor of Nursing
College of Nursing
University of Southern Maine
Portland, Maine

iii

Judy Heggie, RN, MS, DNSc Candidate
Associate Chief of Nursing
   Service/Education
V.A. San Diego Healthcare System
San Diego, California

Elaine M. Hockman, PhD
Research Director
Personalized Nursing Corporation, P.C.
Ann Arbor, Michigan

Bela Horvath, RN, CD
New York, New York

Mary Ireland, RN, PhD
Assistant Professor
College of Nursing
Rutgers, the State University of New Jersey
Newark, New Jersey

Linda Johnston, RN, PhD
University of South Carolina
Aiken, South Carolina

Susan Kun Leddy, RN, PhD
Professor
School of Nursing
Widener University
Chester, Pennsylvania

Mary Madrid, RN, PhD, CCRN
Director of Patient Care
Center for Endovascular Surgery
Beth Israel Medical Center
New York, New York

Violet M. Malinski, RN, PhD
Associate Professor
Hunter Bellevue School of Nursing
Hunter College of the City University of
   New York
New York, New York

Anita Mandl
New York, New York

Katherine E. Matas, RN, PhD
Assistant Professor
College of Nursing
Arizona State University
Tempe, Arizona

Martha A. McNiff, RN, PhD
Nursing Consultant
Psychotherapist
New York, New York

Margaret A. Newman, RN, PhD, FAAN
Professor Emeritus
University of Minnesota
St. Paul, Minnesota

John R. Phillips, RN, PhD
Associate Professor
Division of Nursing
School of Education
New York University
New York, New York

Diane Poulios, RN, MA, OCN
Oncology Nurse Educator
Cancer Center of Saint Barnabas
   Medical Center
Livingston, New Jersey

Pamela G. Reed, RN, PhD, FAAN
Professor and Associate Dean for
   Academic Affairs
College of Nursing
University of Arizona
Tucson, Arizona

Francelyn Reeder, RSM, RN, PhD
Health Science Center
School of Nursing
University of Colorado
Denver, Colorado

Barbara Sarter, RN, FNP, PhD
Associate Professor of Nursing
School of Nursing
University of Southern California
Los Angeles, California

Ann Sullivan Smith, RN, PhD
Director, Nursing Services
Detroit Receiving Hospital and University
   Health Center
Detroit, Michigan

Dorothy Woods Smith, RN, PhD
Associate Professor
College of Nursing
University of Southern Maine
Portland, Maine

Juanita Watson, RN, C, PhD
Assistant Professor of Nursing
Rutgers, the State University of New Jersey
Camden, New Jersey

Tracey A. Woodward, RN, BSN
Consultant in Staff Development
Woodward & Associates
Smyer, Texas

Contents

Foreword

*T*he evolution of the Rogers' Conferences at New York University mirrors the growth of the Science of Unitary Human Beings in many ways. The first conference, held in the early 1980s, grew from the efforts of a small determined group of doctoral students and faculty members who desired a forum where some of their newest thinking and research might be shared more broadly with a group of like-minded nurse scholars. Rogers herself often suggested speakers and topics that usually featured newly completed dissertation research augmented by discussion. In the audience were nurses studying for advance degrees in the New York metropolitan area with some attenders from the deep south and the southwest. Recent conference presenters have included scholars from Brazil, Germany, and the United Kingdom while contributors to this volume live and work in diverse areas throughout the United States.

The early conferences were held every three or four years, and attenders often audiotaped proceedings. Those "pirated tapes" are rare archival resources today. Participants in those early conferences went home with new ideas and insights into this complex, divergent conceptual system; that tradition continues at conferences that are now held every two years.

The intellectual challenges first posed by Rogers in her classes and writings, and taken up by her students and colleagues, have nurtured the development of other thinker/theoreticians like Newman and Parse who regularly attend and participate in the Rogerian Conferences. This book opens with a chapter by Newman in an imaginative creation of a dialogue between Rogers and Bohm that extends the Rogerian legacy (the theme of the most recent conference) of intellectual challenge to the professional discipline of Nursing. Parse, who is one of the most loyal critics of Rogerian Science, has helped Rogerian scholars learn the art of thoughtful critique in the conferences and in her own writing, which has contributed substantially to the development of the science. Chapters toward the end of the book describe ways in which Rogers' seminal thinking is relevant to our consumers and colleagues; a real demonstration of integrality and of power, and certainly consistent with Rogers' own stated belief that the Science of Unitary Human Beings was relevant to all people, not only nurses.

A science is "healthy" as long as it is alive, useful, and developing. The Rogerian Conferences and this book (and previous volumes edited by

Barrett and Madrid & Barrett) are concrete evidence of that fact. Conference presentations and chapters within this volume give ample evidence of the continued lively growth of both the science and the art of nursing within the context of the Science of Unitary Human Beings. Phillips traces the evolution of the science, while Barrett, Leddy, and Fawcett, Cowling, and Reed define and describe, with more precision, conceptual building blocks like power, healthiness, pattern appreciation, and transcendence which clarify and extend understanding of the science. Hanchett, Sarter and Reeder provide further information about and insights into mysticism, suggesting another dimension for exploration within the Science. Researchers like Malinski, Watson, Hastings-Tolsma, Johnston, Gueldner, Carboni, Butcher, and Bultemeier contribute to the methodology and measurement tools consistent with the conceptual system. Younger scholars share their research applications of the conceptual system to timely, real world issues: McNiff examines well-being and life satisfaction among people with long-term healthcare needs. Ireland describes hope among children with AIDS, Watson contributes to understanding of sleep-wake in older women, and Andersen and her colleagues share their findings about practice with an inner city population of substance abusers. While these are certainly not "ivory tower" topics, the nitty-gritty world of daily nursing practice is also addressed by Woodward and Heggie, Horvath, Matas, Poulios and Gold, all of whom can be described as "white shoe" nurses who deliver care to patients/consumers every day, and share their very artful applications of the Science of Unitary Human Beings with readers in this volume.

This treasure chest does offer something for everyone: teacher, practitioner, researcher, consumer, colleague. What else could one expect? Although Rogers' physical body has died, the energy field which is Martha E. Rogers continues to prod, provoke, stimulate, and challenge (and occasionally scold) those nurses and other scholars who know her and listen to what she continues to write, albeit with their collaboration and powerful cooperation.

JOANNE GRIFFIN, RN, PhD

Preface

Let knowledge grow from more to more.
Alfred Tennyson

I have known and loved Martha E. Rogers as a teacher, a mentor, a colleague, and a friend. I first met her in September 1980, at New York University when, as a graduate student, I took the course entitled Science of Man. At that time, she autographed her book *An Introduction to the Theoretical Basis of Nursing* for me with these words, "Best wishes for a very creative future." On October 30, 1993, she wrote her last autograph on the premiere issue of *Visions: The Journal of Rogerian Nursing Science.* It said, "What a wonderful time to be around. Keep going!"

But what did Martha mean when she spoke of a "very creative future" and when she encouraged me and many others to "keep going"? I searched for the answer in writing this preface and was amazed to discover that the answer has been before me from the very first day I met Martha. It was right there in her class handout entitled "Overview of Course:"

> *Many cherished beliefs are becoming obsolete as new knowledge about man and the world pours forth. A universe of open systems, multidimensional energy fields, and dramatic evolutionary innovations presage a future of startling magnitude. The impossible becomes probable. Established laws of nature give way to fresh views. Change is continuous. Sophocles, in ancient Greek literature, has Antigone say, "Is it so difficult, is it shameful to give up positions which, by tomorrow at the latest will no longer be tenable?" Around the turn of the century Sir William Crooks (1832–1910), eminent physicist and chemist, lecturing on the then incredible theories of the composition of matter, introduced his lecture with: "Gentlemen, I know what I am going to tell you is an impossibility according to the established laws of nature. Nevertheless it is true."*
>
> *In this course—Science of Man—you will be introduced to new ways of perceiving man and his environment. (New York University, September 1980)*

Martha knew that the Science of Man, now the Science of Unitary Human Beings, would evolve through a continuous process of increasing knowledge and change. It could never be firmly fixed. She coined new words and discarded former ones. Some took on new meanings. Theories were developed within this framework, research findings shed new light on human/environmental phenomena, and nursing practice was revolutionized.

I believe that what Martha meant by a "very creative future" and to "keep going" was that we should continue to discover new ways to perceive human beings and their environment and contribute to the evolutionary process of growth and change concerning the Science of Unitary Human Beings. Our infinite potential should be used to inspire research, create new theories, new methods of research, and innovative ways to practice the art of nursing in our ever-changing universe.

This book is an attestation that Martha's words, "be creative" and "keep going," were heard and taken to heart by many Rogerian scholars, some of whom presented their work at the Fifth (1994) or Sixth Rogerian Conference (1996) at New York University. Papers submitted from these conferences were selected and revised for inclusion in this publication. Other papers included were submitted by health professionals other than nurses and one by a consumer of healthcare.

This book is organized into five parts. Part One addresses the legacy of Martha E. Rogers and her evolving Science of Unitary Human Beings. Part Two identifies issues of methodology, measurement, and theory testing. Unique, creative methods of research are presented. The development and description of Rogerian tools and their validity and reliability are discussed. The chapter addressing "insights and ideas from 10 years of research" on Barrett's theory of power as knowing participation in change is a valuable resource for researchers. Part Three captures and explores the traditional spirit of the mysticism of the Aborigines of Australia and of Buddhist and Hindu philosophy. Beliefs are compared and contrasted to Rogerian science. Part Four contains a rich repository of Rogerian science-based nursing research from a variety of settings, presenting new ways to perceive human beings and their environment. Part Five demonstrates the innovative and creative application of Rogerian science to practice and to our lives. Physicians speak out on the relevance of the Science of Unitary Human Beings in our 20th-century healthcare system. A client tells us about her experience with Rogerian nursing and a mother shares her experience of childbirth from a Rogerian perspective.

Martha forged a new path in science. Her visionary spirit inspired us to have a never-ending quest for knowledge; she continues to light the way for us to discover new meanings within the Science of Unitary Human Beings. Each contributor in this book presented a creative expression of their research, theory testing, practice, or life experience. It is this creative expression that has great value. As editor, I made every attempt to support this freedom of expression while at the same time maintaining consistency within the framework of Rogerian science.

I thank Elizabeth Ann Manhart Barrett, my dear friend and colleague, for giving me the title for this publication and for her support and valuable editorial assistance. I also thank Allan Graubard, Director of NLN Press for his encouragement and guidance.

Some papers will raise issues that are put forth for scholarly inquiry. We learn and grow from our experience and the scholarly endeavors of others. Martha E. Rogers had a creative vision. Her living presence is with us and her legacy will remain to inspire us to "Keep Going!"

MARY MADRID

Part One

The Legacy of Martha E. Rogers

A Dialogue with Martha Rogers and David Bohm About the Science of Unitary Human Beings

Margaret A. Newman

PREAMBLE

Since I have incorporated David Bohm's theory in much of my writing (Newman, 1986, 1994) and speaking, some people have gotten the impression that my theory of health as expanding consciousness emanated from Bohm's (and other physical scientists') theories. This is not the case, and I would like to set the record straight. My theory evolved from the new paradigm set forth by Martha Rogers. It was first presented in 1978 and published in 1979 (Newman, 1979). When I became familiar with Bohm's work after the publication of his book in 1930, I was delighted that his theory of implicate order, coming from a different disciplinary focus, supported the ideas explicated in my theory regarding disease as a manifestation of the whole and suggested in Rogers' work when she referred to health and illness as a unitary process. I was particularly

*pleased to hear of Martha's interest in revisiting Bohm's theory and her
intuition that the future of nursing science would be enhanced by his
work.*

*I*n the spring of 1994, shortly before her death, Martha Rogers recorded
a message to all of us. One of the things she said was:

*This . . . brings a message for the future that you are going to have to im-
plement.*

And then an aside:

One book I've got to re-read is David Bohm's Implicate Order.

Martha thought that Bohm was still *adding on* consciousness rather than
seeing it as a pattern emerging from the field. Based on her energy field
model, it was clear to her that consciousness was emerging from the field
(Malinski & Barrett, 1994). Bohm died in the fall of 1993, without their
having an opportunity to discuss this phenomenon, but Martha was spec-
ulating that maybe he was sending us a message about it from beyond. I
will revisit the thoughts of David Bohm as they relate to Martha's
thoughts on the Science of Unitary Human Beings.
    In introducing his theory of implicate order, Bohm (1980) said:

*My main concern has been with understanding the nature of reality in
general and of consciousness in particular as a coherent whole, which is
never static or complete, but which is in an unending process of movement and unfoldment. (p. ix)*

He described the problem of *thinking* about movement, that it somehow
comes out seeming static or like a series of static images. So he pursued
the question of *what is the relationship of thinking to reality.* If thought
itself is a part of reality as a whole, how could one part of reality know another? Would this be possible? It is firmly embedded in our tradition that
the one who thinks is separate from the reality that he or she thinks about.

*How are we to think coherently of a single, unbroken, flowing actuality
of existence as a whole, containing both thought . . . and external reality
as we experience it? (Bohm, 1980, p. x)*

In order to understand, we must attend first to what he had to say
about theory. He emphasized that *a world view is the most important*

consideration in science, not the ability to control and predict as some of his fellow physicists and medical scientists would say. Then in order to explain his world view of wholeness and movement, he digresses a bit. He says that it has always been necessary to divide things up, to separate them, in order to make our problems manageable, but this type of activity applies primarily to practical, technical work. If, in our practical work, we tried to deal with the whole all at once, we would be swamped. But this ability to separate ourselves from the environment, and to divide things up, has led to a range of negative, destructive results, one of the most apparent being the pollution of our environment. Humankind lost its awareness of what was being done and extended the process of division beyond the limits within which it works properly.

When our notion of ourselves and the world in which we live (a self-world view) is guided by this mode of thought, then we cease thinking of the divisions as "merely useful or convenient" and begin to see and experience ourselves and our world as constituted of separate fragments:

> *Being guided by a fragmentary self-world view, . . . Man thus obtains an apparent proof of the correctness of his fragmentary self-world view though, of course, he overlooks the fact that it is he himself, acting according to his mode of thought, who has brought about the fragmentation . . . (Bohm, 1980, pp. 2-3)*

Bohm regarded a theory as primarily a form of *insight,* "a way of looking at the world" (p. 4) rather than knowledge of how the world is. He projected that "one may expect *the unending development of new forms of insight.*" (p. 5, emphasis added)

If we are not aware that our theories are ever-changing insights, our vision will be limited. Our experience will be locked into an unchanging view. The belief that theories give true knowledge of reality prevents insights from going beyond existing limitations and changing to meet new facts. This belief also implies that the theories never need to change. This confusion leads us to approach our phenomena of study in terms of more or less fixed and limited forms of thought. (This illustrates how our thinking is a function of our world view.) And, therefore, we continue to confirm the limitations of these thoughts in experience:

> *if we regard our theories as . . . reality . . . , then we will . . . treat these differences and distinctions as divisions, implying separate existence of the various elementary terms appearing in the theory.* We will thus be led to the illusion that the world is actually constituted of separate fragments . . . . *(p. 7, emphasis added)*

Bohm pointed out that some might say that fragmentation is reality, that wholeness is only an ideal. These were familiar charges against Rogers years ago when she first insisted that the human being must be viewed in a unitary way, in indivisible wholeness. Many thought she was asking for more than science could give. But Bohm declared unequivocally:

> *What should be said is that* wholeness is what is real, *and that* fragmentation is the response of the whole to man's action, . . . *which is* shaped by fragmentary thought. . . . *So what is needed is for man to give attention to his habit of fragmentary thought, to be aware of it, and thus bring it to an end. (p. 7, emphasis added)*

We have to give up fragmentary thinking. We have to give up thinking that our theories depict the whole of reality. We have to give up thinking that our theories are final and need never be changed. Bohm went on to say:

> *What is called for is not an* integration *of thought, or a kind of imposed unity, for any such imposed point of view would itself be merely another fragment. Rather, all our different ways of thinking are to be considered as different ways of looking at the one reality . . . The whole . . . is not perceived in any one view but, rather it is grasped only* implicitly . . . . *(pp. 7-8, emphasis in original)*

As Bohm developed his thoughts of wholeness, he was aware of the contradictions between relativistic theory and quantum theory and concentrated on the agreement between the two: the need to view the world as *an undivided whole,* called by Bohm "undivided wholeness in flowing movement," because it is always evolving.

This undivided wholeness echoes Rogers' thoughts that a model of the human being "must affirm the unity of nature" (Rogers, 1970, p. 89), that "Human and environmental fields are . . . contiguous with one another, and coextensive with the universe" (Malinski & Barrett, 1994, p. 223). We cannot separate the person from the environment. We cannot divide up the human being.

> *There is a universal flux that cannot be defined explicitly but which can be known only implicitly"* . . . *mind and matter are not separate substances . . . they are different aspects of one whole and unbroken movement." (Bohm, 1980, p. 11)*

To illustrate the point that various particles in our observed reality are projections of a higher dimensional reality, Bohm suggested that we imagine the projections of a fish tank from two television cameras (A and B) on corresponding screens. The pictures that we see are moving, changing objects that somehow portray the same phenomenon, but neither captures the whole. Each is a limited version of a phenomenon of greater dimensions. In the same way, if our phenomenon of concern is the human being, projections of mind and matter as seen in current literature are limited versions of an indivisible phenomenon of infinite dimensions. They are explications of the underlying implicate whole:

> Our theories are not "descriptions of reality as it is" but, rather, ever-changing forms of insight, which can point to or indicate a reality that is implicit and not describable or specifiable in its totality. (p. 17)

So how do we proceed in theory development? Bohm points out that:

> A major source of fragmentation is indeed the generally accepted presupposition that the process of thought is sufficiently separate from and independent of its content. . . . content and process are not two separately existent things, but rather, they are two aspects of views of one whole movement. (p. 18)
>
> What we have to deal with here is a one-ness of the thinking process and its content, similar in key ways to the oneness of observer and observed . . . . (p. 18)

Bohm cites the ancient Greeks as introducing a concept of measurement that meant inner measure, the proportion of things: "to keep everything in its right measure was regarded as one of the essentials of a good life" (p. 20). It was not measurement against some external standard, but an inner measure of things (a ratio, proportion) that was seen as a key to health:

> The essential reason or ratio of a thing is then the totality of inner proportions in its structure, and in the process in which it forms, maintains itself, and ultimately dissolves. In this view, to understand such ratio is to understand the "innermost being" of that thing. (p. 21)

Ratio is the beginning of pattern. The measure of the innermost being, from a Rogerian point of view, is *pattern* that identifies wholeness.

Bohm proposed that the implicate order be taken as fundamental. This is consistent with Martha's assumption of the unitary nature of the human being. The implicate order applies to both matter and consciousness. We need to come to the notion of a common ground for both.

> If matter and consciousness could in this way be understood together, in terms of the same general notion of order, the way would be opened to comprehending their relationship on the basis of some common ground.

> *Thus we could come to the germ of a new notion of unbroken wholeness, in which consciousness is no longer to be fundamentally separated from matter. (Bohm, 1980, p. 197)*
>
> *In the implicate order we have to say that mind enfolds matter in general and therefore the body in particular. Similarly, the body enfolds not only the mind but also in some sense the entire material universe. (p. 209)*
>
> *So we are led to propose further the more comprehensive, deeper, and more inward actuality is neither mind nor body but rather a yet higher dimensional actuality, which is their common ground and which is of a nature beyond both. (p. 209)*

The common ground is the pattern of the whole. To discover for ourselves the meaning of wholeness, we need to begin all over, to learn afresh. Bohm (1980) asserted:

> *to develop new insight into fragmentation and wholeness requires a creative work event more difficult than that needed to make fundamental new discoveries in science . . . (p. 24)*

Again, he's saying how difficult it is to change our world view. To us as Rogerian scientists, ones who have accepted the paradigm of unitary human beings and who want to extend this knowledge, Bohm has this to say:

> *one who is similar to Einstein [substitute Rogers] in creativity is not the one who imitates Einstein's ideas, nor even the one who applies these ideas in new ways, rather, it is the one who learns from Einstein and then goes on to do something original, which is able to assimilate what is valid in Einstein's work and yet goes beyond this work in qualitatively new ways. (p. 24)*

In response to Martha's ideas, we must learn from her and then go on to do something original. We are developing new methods of study consistent with the Rogerian paradigm. According to Bohm, the creative insight in the field of measure is "the action of the immeasurable." When the insight occurs, it will not come from ideas already contained in the field of measure (the old paradigm) but from the immeasurable, the implicate order. When this happens, the measurable (the explicate) and the immeasurable (the implicate) will be consistent and can be regarded as different ways of measuring the undivided whole:

in the implicate order the totality of existence is enfolded within each re-
gion of space (and time). So whatever part, element, or aspect we may
abstract in thought, this still enfolds the whole and is therefore intrinsi-
cally related to the totality from which it has been abstracted. (p. 172)

This gives us some understanding of how the part can give insight into
the whole. The task of traditional science is to start from the parts and to
derive the wholes. From Bohm:

On the contrary, when one works in terms of the implicate order, one be-
gins with the undivided wholeness of the universe, and the task of sci-
ence is to derive the parts through abstraction from the whole . . .
(p. 179)

In short, we have an order which cannot all be made explicate at once
and which is nevertheless real . . . (p. 183)

What is is always a totality of ensembles, all present together in an or-
derly series of stages of enfoldment and unfoldment, which intermingle
and inter-penetrate each other in principle throughout the whole . . .
(pp. 183–184)

To conclude, the science of unitary human beings is characterized by
undivided wholeness. It is *dynamic, moving.* The observer cannot be separated from the observed. Thinking cannot be separate from the object of
thought. The content is not separate from the process. *Theory is moving*
intuition, evolving insights. The nursing science of unitary human beings
is the study of the moving, intuitive experience of nurses in mutual process with those they serve. The higher order is the pattern of the whole,
which is grasped implicitly, intuitively by seeing the explicate as manifestation of the implicate. It is an advancing idea—like a wave—and as it
unfolds, it incorporates previous knowledge in a new way. Martha's
words heralded Bohm's:

Nursing science is a new product . . . is open-ended; constantly evolving;
never finished. (Rogers, 1968 in Malinski & Barrett, 1994, p. 111)

To actively and creatively participate in realizing the future, whatever it
may hold, demands unparalleled vision, a greatly expanded human com-
passion, the capacity to enjoy uncertainty, and courage to stand up and
be counted; to initiate; to set direction that mankind may benefit. There
is vast promise for those of wisdom, imagination, and daring whose so-
cial concern transcends personal gain and whose integrity does not vac-
illate. (Rogers, 1968 in Malinski & Barrett, 1994, p. 129)

REFERENCES

Bohm, D. (1980). *Wholeness and the implicate order.* London: Routledge & Kegan Paul.

Malinski, V. M., & Barrett, E. A. M. (1994). *Martha E. Rogers: Her life and her work.* Philadelphia: Davis.

Newman, M. A. (1979). *Theory development in nursing.* Philadelphia: Davis.

Newman, M. A. (1986). *Health as expanding consciousness.* St. Louis: Mosby.

Newman, M. A. (1994). *Health as expanding consciousness* (2nd ed.). New York: NLN Press.

Rogers, M. E. (1970). *An introduction to the theoretical basis of nursing.* Philadelphia: Davis.

2

Evolution of the Science of Unitary Human Beings

John R. Phillips

Martha E. Rogers is living; she did *not* die. Her energy field is resonating in the infinite wholeness of the universe, and the universe is her cosmic address. Her living presence is integral with all of us; she is flowing through us, and we are flowing through her. We are infinite energy fields; we can experience her living presence. Rogers has made her presence known and is participating in patterning our environmental field for our unitary well-being.

What is going to happen to the Science of Unitary Human Beings? Rogers (1992) adamantly stated science is open-ended, and believed the Science of Unitary Human Beings will continue to evolve to provide the knowledge for the care of people in an ever-changing world.

You can envision Rogers, smiling and even laughing. Why? Rogers sees the past, present, and future of nursing, the infinite wholeness of nursing in her relative present. Rogers is smiling—she now knows for sure her vision of nursing is true. But, she says, "I see different things now, so expect to see changes in the Science of Unitary Human Beings." Laughing, she says, "So you thought there would be no more changes to my nursing science." Rogers will continue to participate in the evolution of her Science of Unitary Human Beings, through all of us as we study and use it.

As Rogerian scholars experience Rogers' living presence, she will energize them to search for new meanings in the Science of Unitary Human Beings; new meanings for science, nursing science, and all of humankind. She will help us to develop further our belief and faith in the Science of Unitary Human Beings and its use in the science and art of nursing for the care of people, and ultimately for the care of the universe.

Rogers was instrumental for several decades in the development and promulgation of nursing science. She critically examined philosophy and knowledge and transposed them as she evolved her nursing science. It is the responsibility of Rogerian scholars to further elucidate and articulate the philosophy of the Science of Unitary Human Beings so there will be continued evolution of Rogerian science and knowledge.

NURSING PHILOSOPHY

Philosophy is integral to all knowledge. Philosophy has been used in patterning the universe of knowledge to create all of the sciences. This suggests there is an implicate order to the wholeness of the philosophy of the universe of knowledge, whereby there is an integralness of the philosophy and knowledge of all of the sciences. More specifically, there is an implicate order to the wholeness of nursing philosophy and knowledge (see Figure 2.1).

Philosophy gives a broad perspective to nursing and to nursing science. In fact, it serves as the ground for the actual and potential knowledge that can be created/discovered. The power of nurse scholars to generate nursing knowledge and to develop nursing science becomes evident as nursing philosophy is articulated and used. An understanding of the place of philosophy in nursing is essential for a science-based practice.

One of the major tasks for nurses is to identify the philosophy that serves as the ground for nursing. There needs to be greater clarity in the identification of the basic tenets of nursing philosophy. Through the specification of nursing science, nurses can further explicate nursing philosophy and knowledge from the universe of philosophy and knowledge. This is essential so nurses can enrich nursing philosophy and create new knowledge to comprehend their own reality and the reality of their clients.

One of the distinctive attributes of nursing philosophy is the coherence it gives to nursing science. Philosophy enables nurses to identify the patterns of knowledge in nursing science. Multiple patterns of knowledge

Figure 2.1   Relation of Philosophy and Nursing Philosophy
and Science for Practice

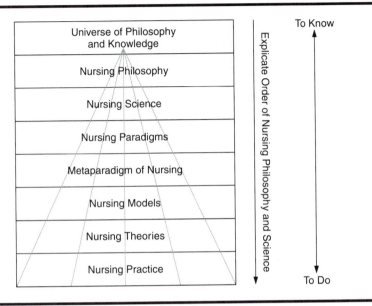

need to be identified/created to give substance to nursing science. A variety of philosophies and patterns of knowledge give diversity to nursing science, and ultimately enhance the creative, innovative process of nurses. There is resonance among the patterns of knowledge giving unity in the diversity of nursing science.

Nurses' identification/creation of philosophical patterns of nursing knowledge is not a linear process. Carper's (1992) patterns of knowing provide for a mutual process of the nurse and the environment so nurses can understand the wholeness of the knowledge of nursing science. Carper presents these patterns of knowing as empirics, the science of nursing; ethics, the component of moral knowledge; esthetics, the art of nursing; and personal knowledge. These patterns of knowing pervade all of nursing science to help nurses create nursing philosophy and knowledge for practice. It is nurses' pattern recognition, moving beyond facts and isolated theories, that accelerates the explication of nursing philosophy and knowledge.

Nursing philosophy and science are given greater specification through nursing paradigms (see Figure 2.1). Nursing paradigms give specific philosophical and knowledge bases for the development of the metaparadigm of nursing, which is used to create nursing models. When one considers nursing models at the paradigm level, one must realize the boundaries placed upon a nursing model by its philosophical ground. As Koziol-McLain and Maeve (1993) state, "The realities of nursing practice will always go beyond even the most comprehensive of theories" (p. 79). Moreover, these paradigms set the parameters for nursing practices to provide answers to practice questions.

Two prominent sets of nursing paradigms are Parse's (1987) totality and simultaneity paradigms and Newman, Sime, and Corcoran-Perry's (1991) particulate-deterministic, interactive-integrative, and unitary-transformative perspectives. The details of these paradigms can be found in the works of the cited authors, as well as in Fawcett (1993). Briefly, Parse's totality paradigm sees people as parts, while the simultaneity paradigm sees people as wholes. For Newman et al. (1991), the particulate-deterministic perspective sees clients in practice settings as reducible and predictable in linear and causal relationships. This contrasts with the interactive-integrative perspective where clients are seen as multiple, inter-related parts and reality is multidimensional and contextual. The unitary-transformative, however, transcends both of the other two perspectives to see clients as wholes, where there is an emphasis on pattern.

The significance of the unitary-transformative perspective for the Science of Unitary Human Beings is recognized when one sees how Carper's patterns of knowing are related to Newman et al.'s (1991) statement: "Knowledge is personal, involves pattern recognition, and is a function of both viewer and the phenomenon viewed. The subject matter includes thoughts, values, feelings, choices and purpose" (p. 4). Carper (1992) in discussing the relationship of the patterns of knowing states, "Such interdependence more accurately reflects the complexity and richness of nursing practice and the kinds of knowledge required in making clinical judgments" (p. 77). Thus, it is understandable how Newman et al. can state that "a unitary-transformative perspective is essential for full explication of the discipline" (p. 5).

Each nursing paradigm gives a specific view of person, environment, health, and nursing, which, collectively, are known as the metaparadigm of nursing (Fawcett, 1995) (see Figure 2.1). The metaparadigm concepts are used in the creation of nursing models. It is the models that provide the theories for practice and provide the base for generating theories from practice. Here, we need to keep in mind that theories have the same philosophical base as the science from which they were derived. Thus, there is a continuous flow of the universe of philosophy through nursing philosophy, science, paradigms, metaparadigms, models, theories, and ultimately to nursing practice (see Figure 2.1).

This process of philosophy in tandem with the process of nursing knowledge development provides for a science-based practice. As shown in Figure 2.1, this involves the explicate order, the unfolding of nursing philosophy and science to reveal knowledge for practice. There is movement from "to know," a knowledge base, the science of nursing, to "to do," nursing practice, the art of nursing. This certainly conforms to Rogers' (1992) belief that nursing science is a body of knowledge and the art of nursing is the imaginative and creative use of this knowledge.

IMPLICATIONS OF PHILOSOPHY FOR THE EVOLUTION OF THE SCIENCE OF UNITARY HUMAN BEINGS

The brief presentation of the relationship of philosophy to nursing science, and eventually its flow to nursing practice, was done to draw attention to the significance of philosophy in the evolution of the Science of Unitary Human Beings. Rogerian scholars have the responsibility and obligation to enrich the philosophy for the unitary nature, the wholeness, of Rogers' Science of Unitary Human Beings. The significance of Rogerian philosophy is illustrated in Figure 2.2.

Rogers (1970) addressed the issue of scientific knowledge, some people would say philosophy, in the original presentation of her Science of Unitary Human Beings in her book *An Introduction to the Theoretical Basis of Nursing*. Other authors (e.g., Carboni, 1991; Hanchett, 1992; Reeder, 1993; Sarter, 1988, 1989) have addressed philosophical issues as related to Rogers' Science of Unitary Human Beings. These authors, as well as others such as Maliniski (1990), have identified the similarities and differences of specific philosophies and scientific perspectives to

Figure 2.2   Relation of Philosophy of Science of Unitary Human Beings, Science of Unitary Human Beings and Nursing Practice

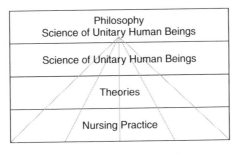

Rogers' nursing science. These authors indicate a need for a more in-depth presentation of the philosophy for Rogers' nursing science. Further identification of the philosophical tenets will help in the evolution of the Science of Unitary Human Beings, rather than just a repetition of Rogers' descriptions of the basic elements of her nursing science.

Even Rogers (1992) stated, "The science of nursing was arrived at by the creative synthesis of facts and ideas and is an emergent, a new product" (p. 28). Rogers consistently emphasized in her writings that her nursing science was a new product. In fact, she says, "The science of unitary human beings has not derived from one or more of the basic sciences. Neither has it come out of a vacuum. It flows instead in novel ways from a multiplicity of knowledge, from many sources, to create a kaleidoscope of potentialities" (p. 28). Since the Science of Unitary Human Beings is a new product, then one can question the relevancy of other philosophies or sciences, as indicated by Rogers, for the Science of Unitary Human Beings, or for the interpretation of its philosophical tenets. One can conclude, however, that a philosophy and a knowledge base specific to the Science of Unitary Human Beings are needed for its continued evolution.

The challenge for Rogerian scholars, then, is to further elucidate the philosophy of the Science of Unitary Human Beings. The first step might be to look at the words "unitary human beings." Rogers is not using the word "unitary" as found in any of the other philosophies or sciences, even though on the surface they appear to be similar. Even though Rogers advocated the use of the general language dictionary to define words, the dictionaries do not present the philosophical base for them.

The elucidation and articulation of a Rogerian philosophy requires Rogerian scholars to analyze Rogers' writings within the context of the universe of philosophy and knowledge to elicit the defining attributes of the concept of unitary human beings and its philosophical base. This process requires creative and imaginative thinking that goes beyond the writings of Rogers to uncover and give interpretation of the philosophical meaning of what she intended when she coined "unitary human beings." Other Rogerian scholars must do a thoughtful scrutiny of these interpretations to assure these new meanings/ideas are true to Rogerian science. Rogerian scholars cannot afford to take any false paths in the continued evolution of Rogers' nursing science. However, we must be sure our cautious approach does not stifle the commitment to evolve the Science of Unitary Human Beings in creative and innovative ways. As was stated by Kaku (1994), "science would be sterile and empty, and progress nonexistent, without dreamers" (p. 16).

The essential task of looking at the philosophical base for the concept of unitary human beings is not an isolated one, but must take into consideration simultaneously the basic elements of Rogers' Science of Unitary Human Beings (see Figure 2.3). Rogerian scholars must always recognize that the basic elements are integral to the philosophy of the Science of Unitary Human Beings, and all are changing together.

Rogerian scholars must do similar thoughtful analyses of the postulates of the Science of Unitary Human Beings. These postulates emerged from Rogers' (1970) original five assumptions presented in *An Introduction to the Theoretical Basis of Nursing*. Since the words *building blocks* conveyed hierarchy and linearity, Rogers chose the word *postulate* to convey a scientific perspective consistent with her nonlinear nursing science. Rogers transposed philosophy and knowledge from other sciences to create her own meanings of the postulates of openness, energy fields, pattern, and pandimensionality. However, through her writings we know, both conceptually and intuitively, that her meanings of these postulates are different from those found in the literature. Rogers indicates that even though Einstein's ideas of four-dimensionality are germane, her meaning of pandimensionality is not the same.

Rogers (1992) defined pattern as "the distinguishing characteristic of an energy field perceived as a single wave" (p. 29). Rogerian scholars have the responsibility to enrich Rogers' philosophical and theoretical base for her concept of pattern. Questions they might pose are, "What is the purpose of pattern?, Why is pattern a distinguishing characteristic?, What are the attributes of a Rogerian perspective of pattern?"

Too, Rogers' idea of a "single wave" is not the same as the linear wave found in physics. Many people use the traditional physics' view in trying to understand her single wave. A philosophical question Rogerian scholars might ask is, "What is a pandimensional single wave, and what are its attributes?" Questions of this nature are being pursued by doctoral

Figure 2.3   Relation of Philosophy and Basic Elements of the
Science of Unitary Human Beings

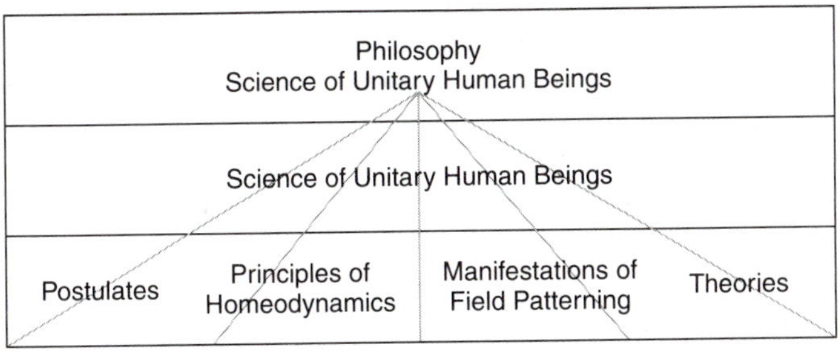

students at New York University. One student is doing a philosophical study of the evolution of the concept of energy. The generation of such knowledge will help more people to appreciate the elegance of Rogers' Science of Unitary Human Beings, and the beauty of its abstractness.

Philosophical and theoretical knowledge of the concept of unitary human beings and the postulates is essential to a full understanding of the principles of homeodynamics. These three principles—helicy, resonancy, and integrality—are concerned with the nature and process of change in pattern. Rogers' refinement of these principles over the years is discussed by Maliniski (1994) in the book *Martha E. Rogers: Her Life and Her Work.* Moreover, Malinski does a thoughtful analysis of other changes in Rogers' Science of Unitary Human Beings.

One of Rogers' most profound changes was the replacement of probabilistic with unpredictable in the principle of helicy. Even though Rogers (1992) has briefly discussed this change and stated, "new knowledge supports it" (p. 32), it is also clear that this new knowledge does not have the same meaning for unpredictability as she is using it. A word of caution is needed here. We all know that contemporary science is changing rapidly, and that many of its basic ideas appear to be similar to Rogers' Science of Unitary Human Beings. In fact, Rogers and Rogerian scholars have used this contemporary science to discuss Rogerian nursing science. However, when the basic assumptions of this contemporary science are evaluated, you will still find, as stated by Rogers, the traditional view of linearity, prediction, and cause and effect. Therefore, the contemporary views must be transposed into a Science of Unitary Human Beings perspective before they are used, as suggested by Walker and Avant (1995) in their book on theory construction.

As the philosophy of the Science of Unitary Human Beings is elucidated, which requires going far beyond these brief suggestions, Rogers' full meaning of unpredictable will become more manifest. Simultaneously, new research methods will have to be created by Rogerian scholars to study the unpredictable flow of energy, the dynamic, ever-changing patterning of human and environmental fields, rather than the static slices of energy captured by many of our current research methods. The generation of such knowledge will revolutionize all views of the universe, similar to Einstein's theory of relativity. The philosophical tenets and knowledge that emerge from such research will accelerate the evolution of the Science of Unitary Human Beings, and give new meanings and interpretations to the other sciences, even the arts and humanities as they portray the diverse manifestations of human beings.

All of us know of Rogers' distaste for anything that is linear. This is the reason she eventually deleted the phrase "the nature and direction of" from the current definition of the principle of helicy. Frequently, Rogers has been asked what she intended to do about the apparent linearity in the principle of resonancy, "Continuous change from lower to higher frequency wave patterns in human and environmental fields" (Rogers, 1992, p. 31). Her typical reply was, "I'm thinking about it," which meant she would eventually have the answer. On many occasions, people have discussed the principle of resonancy with Rogers with the hopes of an insight as to how it should be changed, or if it should be changed. This may be the opportune time to experience the living presence of Rogers to learn the answer, especially since she is experiencing the infinite wholeness of nursing, particularly her Science of Unitary Human Beings, where *everything* is manifest in her relative present.

However, until we have this experience, the issue of linearity with the principle of resonancy can be considered simultaneously with Rogers' Manifestations of Field Patterning in Unitary Human Beings (see Appendix). Rogers deleted several manifestations of field patterning as she made changes in her Science of Unitary Human Beings over the years. At one time the words "*From"* and "*In the Direction of"* appeared above the three columns of manifestations. Even though some people see the three columns as linear, we must, however, be sure this linearity does not appear in our Rogerian scholarly writing and research.

Suggestions have been made to place all the manifestations in one column in random order to get rid of what appears to be linearity (Phillips, 1989). Then, people have the potential to experience these manifestations relative to the wave frequency diversity of their mutual human field pattern and environmental field pattern process. It is this relative frequency diversity patterning that is important in understanding what Rogers means by lower to higher frequency. The manifestations can be seen as a resonating low-high frequency diversity of field pattern involving the mutual flow of human-environment energy. When a hyphen is placed between lower frequency and higher frequency, there is a single resonating low-high frequency taking place that manifests as higher frequency diversity of pattern. As indicated in this statement, this process involves all three principles of homeodynamics: higher frequency, innovative, unpredictable increasing diversity that emerges from the mutual process. For example, as indicated in Figure 2.4, person one can have a resonating wave frequency pattern manifesting time experienced as slower and time experienced as faster, while person two can have a resonating wave frequency pattern that manifests time experienced as slower and timelessness. Within this context, one could postulate that people are not really going from lower to higher frequency in a linear way, but are using their potential resonating wave frequency to create

Figure 2.4   Nonlinear View of Manifestations of Field Patterning in Unitary Human Beings

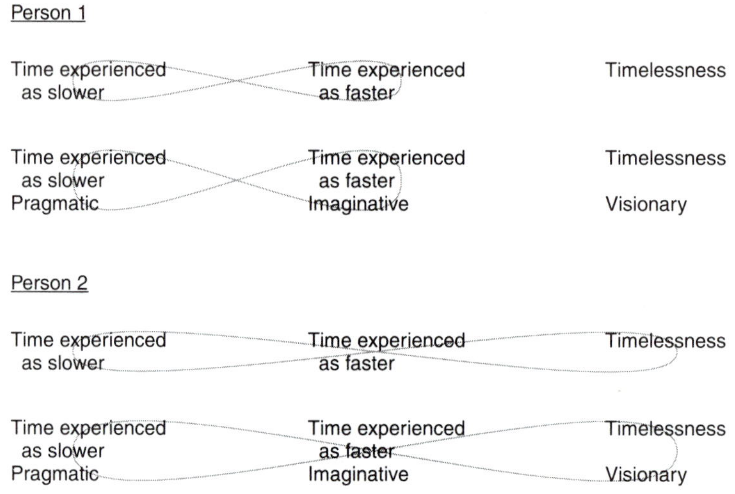

Person 1

Time experienced as slower — Time experienced as faster — Timelessness

Time experienced as slower / Time experienced as faster — Timelessness
Pragmatic — Imaginative — Visionary

Person 2

Time experienced as slower — Time experienced as faster — Timelessness

Time experienced as slower — Time experienced as faster — Timelessness
Pragmatic — Imaginative — Visionary

increasing higher frequency diversity of pattern. Could this not be one possible interpretation of what Rogers means by the principle of resonancy?

With this interpretation, it is possible that people who can hear microwaves (and some people can!) would have a higher frequency diversity of field pattern than those people whose hearing does not include microwaves. One can say that the experiencing of microwaves, which is currently believed, by some people, to be an inaudible low frequency wave, involves increasing frequency diversity of field pattern that emerges from the mutual human field and environmental field process. The broadening of hearing to include lower frequency sound waves negates the traditional linear concept of going from lower to higher frequency wave patterns.

Furthermore, a person's field pattern can increase in diversity when two manifestations are considered simultaneously, where each manifestation has its resonating low-high frequency (see Figure 2.4). This would signify a resonating low-high frequency for two manifestations, rather than strictly going from lower to higher frequency. For example, person one can have a resonating frequency rhythm that involves experiencing time as slow and experiencing time as fast and be pragmatic and imaginative. Person two can have a resonating frequency rhythm for experiencing time as slow and timelessness and be pragmatic and visionary. When looking at the wave frequency diversity pattern of an individual, the integral nature of all manifestations needs to be considered rather than just one or two manifestations to understand the unitary nature of a person. Such a process is inherent in Marie Hastings-Tolsma's (1992) theory of diversity of human field pattern and the instrument she developed to measure diversity of human field pattern.

Once we have lateral thinking of this nature, we will be able to solve what seems to be a paradox of lower to higher frequency wave patterns. Along with further explication of the philosophy of the Science of Unitary Human Beings, we can create new theories that explain and describe this resonating change so we can better understand the increasing wave frequency diversity of pattern. It is this resonating change in pattern diversity that has significance for nursing practice.

IMPLICATIONS FOR NURSING PRACTICE

The further explication of the philosophy of the Science of Unitary Human Beings will help Rogerian scholars to be originators in the creation of new patterns of knowledge, more specifically, nursing knowledge. These patterns of knowledge give insights that help nurses create new ways to care for people. The continued evolution of Rogers' abstract nursing science will open up new vistas for nursing practice. As noted by Silva (1986), "Abstractness has power," and "In abstractness one can be creative, one can dare to imagine beyond the bounds of traditional reality" (p. 9). This is especially true for Rogerian practice.

Many of our current nursing practices will become obsolete in the future, similar to the obsolescence of past nursing practices. In fact, in the future a lot of our present nursing knowledge and practices will be placed in the archives of nursing as being archaic.

There are many insights that come with the evolution of the Science of Unitary Human Beings. One new insight of significance is the relation of the human energy field and the physical body. There are many manifestations of the human field pattern that can be seen, while others cannot be seen. From a Rogerian perspective, the physical body is only one of many manifestations of the human field pattern. Essentially, each person can say, "I am a human energy field that can manifest a physical body" (Phillips, 1991, p. 143). From a Rogerian perspective, the physical body and the human energy field are integral with each other. This is in sharp contrast to the traditional view of people as being composed of parts, such as the biopsychosocial. The primary focus of the composite view is on how well each part is functioning, sometimes in isolation from other parts, with no recognition of a human energy field.

Recognizing the dangers of oversimplification, a brief sketch can be given for two of the many views of human beings (see Figure 2.5), as related to people's experience of health. The traditional view basically sees human beings as machines, which is based on the assumptions of mechanism and reductionism. The human being consists of parts, with each discipline giving its specific labels to these parts. The totality of the human being consists of a summation or addition of these parts.

All a person needs to do is keep these parts functioning well. During the life process, these parts gradually wear out, and eventually the human being dies. Medicine and some nursing models use such a view where emphasis is given to signs and symptoms of disease/illness. This is usually done through the lens of cause and effect, with a seeking for the cause so the effect can be dealt with effectively. Once the cause is determined, treatment modalities such as drugs, surgery, and radiation are given to bring about changes in the health/illness status of the person. There is a desire for homeostasis, better known as equilibrium.

Today, the use of highly sophisticated technology is frequently used to give greater focus to body parts, even to the point where there is concern for parts of the parts of a human being. All of this is for prediction and control, with the purpose of prevention or cure of disease/illness to create health for the person. The traditional view includes multiple perspectives of health, where one extreme is absence of disease. Toward the other end of the continuum, one must have the ability to adapt to stressors.

An opposite view of mechanism and reductionism is a unitary view that comes from the science of unitary human beings (see Figure 2.5). In a science of wholeness, human beings are irreducible energy fields; in other words there are no parts. There is an understanding that human beings have an awareness of their wholeness and of their integrality with the environment, where both change together in a dynamic way. Since the change process is mutual, causation is not relative to their life process. Since they are pandimensional, they are not confined to a linear, three-dimension world but can flow with the infinite nature of a nonlinear universe.

Change is manifest as innovative growing diversity of field pattern, in which people participate knowingly. Patterning—healing modalities are used in patterning the environment. Thus, since the human field and the environment are integral, people participate in patterning their own field. Most important is the idea that change in pattern is unpredictable, which is contrary to the prediction and control found in mechanism and reductionism. During the whole change process, a person's unitary well-being emerges from this patterning process.

Figure 2.5　Two Views of Human Beings: Unitary and Traditional

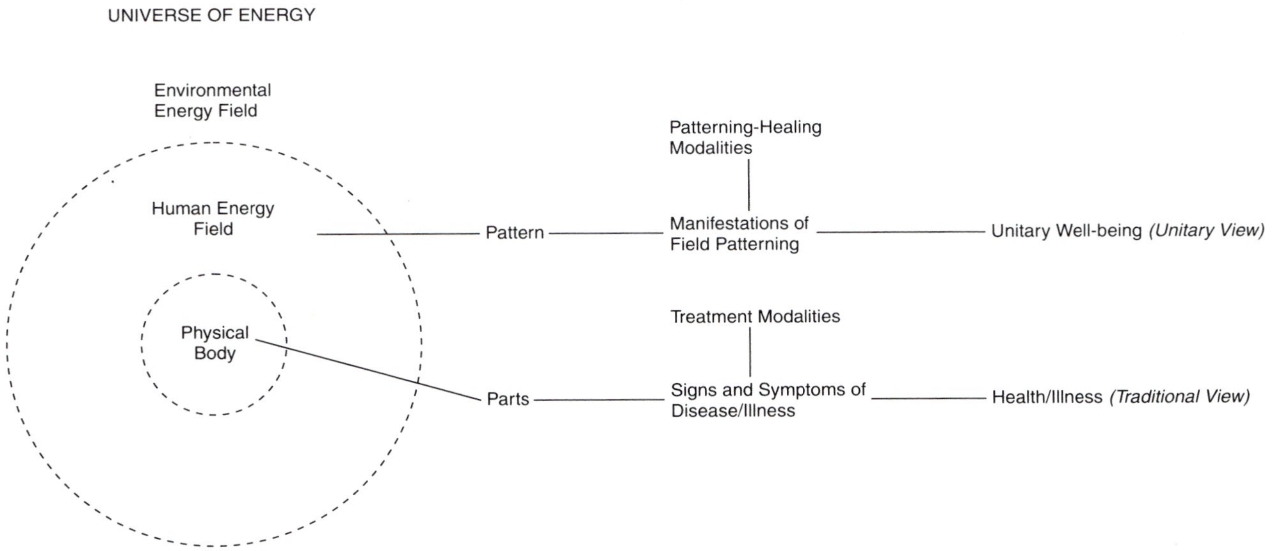

UNIVERSE OF ENERGY

Environmental
Energy Field

Human Energy
Field

Physical
Body

Pattern —————— Manifestations of —————— Unitary Well-being (*Unitary View*)
　　　　　　　　Field Patterning

Patterning-Healing
Modalities

Parts —————— Signs and Symptoms of —————— Health/Illness (*Traditional View*)
　　　　　　　Disease/Illness

Treatment Modalities

Figure 2.6 Process for Unitary Well-Being

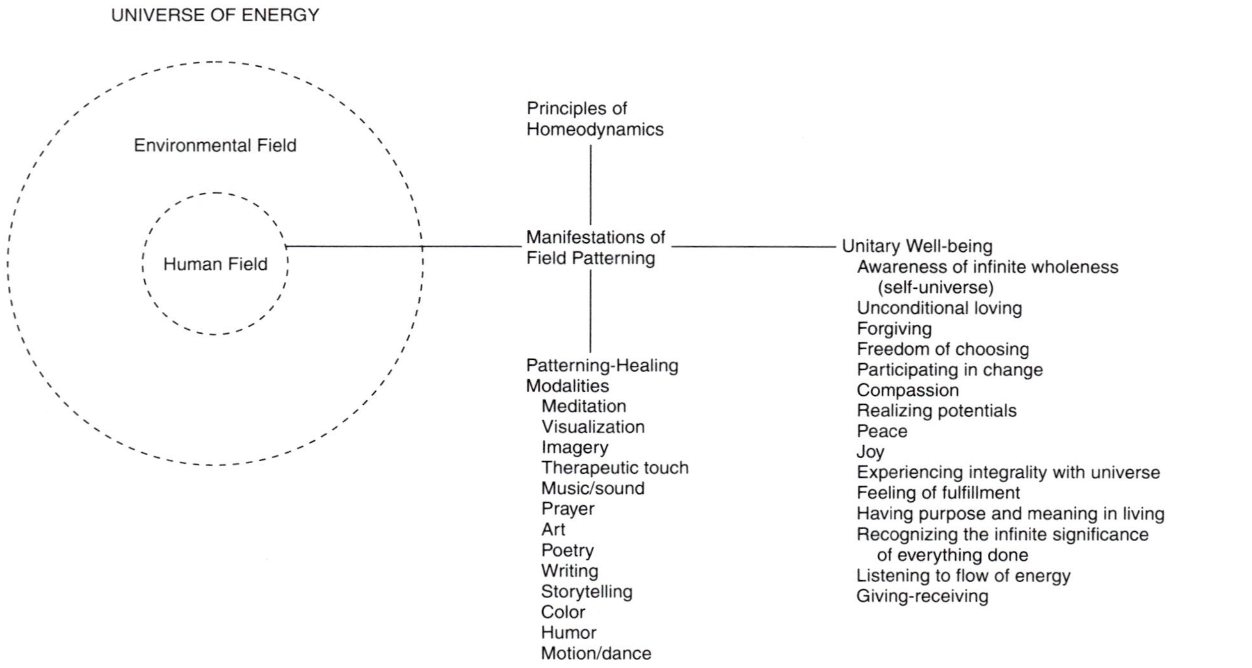

UNIVERSE OF ENERGY

Environmental Field

Human Field

Principles of Homeodynamics

Manifestations of Field Patterning

Patterning-Healing Modalities
Meditation
Visualization
Imagery
Therapeutic touch
Music/sound
Prayer
Art
Poetry
Writing
Storytelling
Color
Humor
Motion/dance

Unitary Well-being
Awareness of infinite wholeness
    (self-universe)
Unconditional loving
Forgiving
Freedom of choosing
Participating in change
Compassion
Realizing potentials
Peace
Joy
Experiencing integrality with universe
Feeling of fulfillment
Having purpose and meaning in living
Recognizing the infinite significance
    of everything done
Listening to flow of energy
Giving-receiving

The question arises as to how nurses participate in a person's well-being. The patterning-healing process for unitary well-b(shown in Figure 2.6. To emphasize again, all manifestations of fie terning emerge from the mutual human field and environmenta. ield process. Rogers' (1992) principles of homeodynamics are used to explain and describe these manifestations to understand the changes in pattern. Once these pattern changes are understood, patterning-healing modalities can be used to help people experience unitary well-being. Barrett's (1990) theory of power is integral to this patterning-healing process.

The openness of the human-environment gives people the ability to participate knowingly in their becoming. Once there is awareness of field manifestations, people are free to make choices, using their own philosophy and values. According to Barrett (1990), people's awareness and choices give the freedom to act intentionally to participate in creating change. There is freedom of action where there are no boundaries to the flow of energy to experience their hopes and dreams. As Curtin (1979) said, when we are open to and supportive of people's decision making, we may be performing our greatest service to them and their family. One could say this is helping people to experience unitary well-being.

Some examples of patterning-healing modalities and attributes of unitary well-being can be found in Figure 2.6. Knowledge of pattern and well-being takes us beyond the confines of the physical body. As Talbot (1991) stated, the reason illnesses often recur is that medicine currently treats only the physical body, and not the human energy field. This idea is echoed by Huffington (1994) who states, "Since life is more than physical, healing must be more than physical too" (p. 110). With continued evolution of Rogers' Science of Unitary Human Beings, people will be able to experience the flow of energy, even to "listen" to the flow of energy to manifest their implicate potentials and their unitary well-being.

CONCLUSION

Rogers is living. The Science of Unitary Human Beings is alive and will continue to evolve as people generate new knowledge. As Rogerian scholars and futurists, we will keep nursing alive in a rapidly changing universe. We have the responsibility to participate knowingly in changing the health care system so all people can have optimum unitary well-being.

It is through the use of Rogers' Science of Unitary Human Beings that we can participate in making manifest the infinite wholeness of nursing. We know there is a future nursing practice we can only dream about, yet we "know" it will become a reality. It is up to us to create the knowledge and practice that help people to manifest their unitary well-being. We must be willing to let Rogers take us beyond the traditional medicine or health care we are experiencing today. Are we willing to take this patterning-healing journey for the unitary well-being of humankind and the universe?

REFERENCES

Barrett, E. A. M. (1990). Health patterning with clients in private practice. In E. A. M. Barrett (Ed.), *Visions of Rogers' science-based nursing* (pp. 105-115). New York: National League for Nursing.

Carboni, J. T. (1991). A Rogerian theoretical tapestry. *Nursing Science Quarterly, 4,* 130-136.

Carper, B. A. (1992). Philosophical inquiry in nursing: An application. In J. F. Kikuchi & H. Simmons (Eds.), *Philosophic inquiry in nursing* (pp. 71-80). Newbury Park, CA: Sage.

Curtin, L. L. (1979). The nurse as advocate: A philosophical foundation for nursing. *Advances in Nursing Science, 1*(3), 1-10.

Fawcett, J. (1993). *Analysis and evaluation of nursing theories.* Philadelphia: Davis.

Fawcett, J. (1995). *Analysis and evaluation of conceptual models of nursing* (3rd ed.). Philadelphia: Davis.

Hanchett, E. S. (1992). Concepts from eastern philosophy and Rogers' science of unitary human beings. *Nursing Science Quarterly, 5,* 164-170.

Hastings-Tolsma, M. T. (1992). The relationship of diversity of human field pattern to risk taking and time experience: An investigation of Rogers' principles of homeodynamics. Unpublished doctoral dissertation, New York University, New York.

Huffington, A. (1994). *The fourth instinct: The call of the soul.* New York: Simon & Schuster.

Kaku, M. (1994, June 19). Science would get nowhere without dreamers. *New York Times,* p. 16.

Koziol-McLain, J., & Maeve, M. K. (1993). Nursing theory in perspective. *Nursing Outlook, 41,* 99-110.

Malinski, V. M. (1990). The meaning of a progressive world view in nursing: Rogers' science of unitary human beings. In N. L. Chaska (Ed.), *The nursing profession: Turning points* (pp. 237-244). St. Louis: Mosby.

Malinski, V. M. (1994). Highlights in the evolution of nursing science: Emergence of the science of unitary human beings. In V. M. Malinski & E. A. M. Barrett, *Martha E. Rogers: Her life and her work* (pp. 197-204). Philadelphia: Davis.

Newman, M. A., Sime, A. M., & Corcoran-Perry, S. A. (1991). The focus of the discipline of nursing. *Advances in Nursing Science, 14*(1), 1-6.

Parse, R. R. (1987). *Nursing science: Major paradigms, theories, and critiques.* Philadelphia: Saunders.

Phillips, J. R. (1989). Science of unitary human beings: Changing research perspectives. *Nursing Science Quarterly, 2,* 57-60.

Phillips, J. R. (1991). Human field research. *Nursing Science Quarterly, 4,* 142-143.

Reeder, F. (1993). The science of unitary human beings and interpretive human science. *Nursing Science Quarterly, 6,* 13-24.

Rogers, M. E. (1970). *An introduction to the theoretical basis of nursing.* Philadelphia: Davis.

Rogers, M. E. (1992). Nursing science and the space age. *Nursing Science Quarterly, 5,* 27-34.

Sarter, B. (1988). Philosophical sources of nursing theory. *Nursing Science Quarterly, 1,* 52-59.

Sarter, B. (1989). Some critical philosophical issues in the science of unitary human beings. *Nursing Science Quarterly, 2,* 74-78.

Silva, M. C. (1986). Research testing nursing theory: State of the art. *Advances in Nursing Science, 9*(1), 1-11.

Talbot, M. (1991). *The holographic universe.* New York: HarperCollins.

Walker, L. O., & Avant, K. C. (1995). *Strategies for theory construction in nursing* (3rd ed.). Norwalk, CT: Appleton & Lange.

Part Two

Rogerian Science Research Methodology, Measurement, and Theory Testing

3

Power as Knowing Participation in Change: Theoretical, Practice, and Methodological, Issues, Insights, and Ideas

Elizabeth Ann Manhart Barrett, Cynthia Caroselli, Anne Sullivan Smith, and Dorothy Woods Smith

*I*n this chapter, we will discuss the Rogerian power theory as the conceptual base for a number of research studies and their practice implications. The group acknowledges with appreciation the substantive work of other researchers who have likewise engaged in the ongoing development and testing of this Rogerian power theory. Numbers will be used to introduce the dialogue questions that were developed by the authors as a group.

OVERVIEW OF POWER THEORY

DR. BARRETT: Elaborating Rogers' (1970, 1990) postulate that humans can participate knowingly in change, power, from a Rogerian perspective, is the capacity to participate knowingly in the nature of change characterizing the continuous patterning of the human and environmental fields. The observable, measurable pattern manifestations of power are awareness, choices, freedom to act intentionally, and involvement in creating change (Barrett, 1986).

Power as knowing participating is being aware of what one is choosing to do, feeling free to do it, and doing it intentionally. Awareness and freedom to act intentionally guide participation in choices. Power is freedom to make aware choices regarding involvement in life changes, including health promoting situations. People actualize selected potentials and participate in creating their reality by being aware, making choices, feeling free to act on their intentions and orchestrating desired changes (Barrett, 1983, 1986, 1989, 1990a, 1990b).

The integral nature of the four power dimensions constitutes the individual's unique power profile which is not static, nonlinear, and varies based on the changing nature of the human and environmental field patterning. Fluctuations reflect: (1) the nature of the awareness of experiences; (2) the type of choices made; (3) the degree to which freedom to act intentionally is experienced; and (4) the type of involvement in creating specific changes.

Theoretical Issues

DR. BARRETT: **1. How can the power theory be further developed?**
    Qualitative research is one way to validate, expand, or revise this theory of power. Dr. Anne Sullivan Smith (1993) completed one of the first Rogerian qualitative studies on power.

DR. A. S. SMITH: Silva and Sorrell (1992) identified three alternative approaches to verifying nursing theory: critical reasoning, description of personal experiences, and application to nursing practice. My study used the second approach (A. Smith, 1993). I interviewed 15 persons who had participated in an organized cardiac rehabilitation program and 18 who had not participated. I asked them how they had made changes after experiencing a cardiac problem, that is, changes in their diets, exercise, activity routines, patterns of work and relaxation, quitting smoking, and any other things they wanted to share about their experience.

There were eight themes drawn from the information of those who participated in a program. They found that it was important to have healthcare professionals reminding them of the importance of attending. Structure and environment at the rehabilitation center helped them to change. Support from family members and comments from the rehab program staff helped them to make lifestyle changes. They also said they "just do it"; they just made the changes.

Six themes were drawn from the interview information of the 18 who did not participate in an organized cardiac rehabilitation program. They said they talked with their doctors about decisions regarding surgery and medical treatments. They reported that having a support system of family and friends made a difference in their recovery.

The themes that were drawn from the interviews were compared with Barrett's dimensions of power. Expressions of their experience with making health changes support Barrett's description of the four dimensions of power as knowing participation in change. Themes of those who did not participate in a structured rehab program were more congruent with the power dimensions than the themes of the structured program participants. This reminds me of Dr. Rogers' message in Malinski's book regarding the Doubting Thomases we meet. Perhaps they know something we don't! We need to learn to listen to those who hear a different drummer.

DR. BARRETT: It will be interesting to see how Howard Butcher's Unitary Human Field Pattern Portrait Methodology, Judith Carboni's Rogerian Process of Inquiry, Richard Cowling's Pattern Appreciation Case Study Method, and other new methods will lend themselves to further development of the power theory. How else can the power theory be further developed using qualitative or quantitative methods?

DR. CAROSELLI: Power and change are inescapable phenomena associated with unitary human beings. Invariably, power and change are associated with conflict, as people become aware of differences in each other's values, beliefs, and goals. As we evolve through healthcare reform, a potentially fruitful line of inquiry is that related to formulating a theoretical approach to conflict that is grounded in the Barrettian power theory. This inquiry could involve an examination or exploration for the operational indicators of conflict, a tool to measure conflict, an investigation of the relationship of power and conflict, and finally, a Barrettian approach to conflict resolution that moves beyond positional bargaining, and domination and submission.

DR. BARRETT: **2. Of the four dimensions of power, are there some dimensions that are more critical than others? In other words, do any of the concepts make a greater difference in power than the others?**

To begin with, they are all integral with each other. That mix of the four dimensions is what I call the *power profile*. Individually, they don't represent power; they represent separate phenomena. Knowing everything there is to know about each of the four dimensions doesn't tell us anything about power. Rather, we are required to describe the integral nature of all four when we describe power. However, as we look at how the dimensions fluctuate in quality and quantity, then we can talk about differences. I believe that in different situations, various dimensions may seem primary, the most critical at that time. Dorothy, you have used the theory in practice rather extensively, what is your view?

DR. D. W. SMITH: The question is a provocative one. As I ponder the nature of patterns that are identifiable as unique as well as inextricable from the whole, I think of the dimensions of awareness and feeling free to act intentionally as representing knowing, and involvement in creating change and choices as manifestations of participation. Power is different from the sum of the dimensions.

The theory of power seemed to describe some of what I saw in many polio survivors. I tested the relationship of power and spirituality in a national study of 252 people, 172 polio survivors and 80 people who had not had polio or any other similar or life-threatening illness. Findings supported a positive relationship between power and spirituality ($r = .34, p < .005$), and that polio survivors manifested greater spirituality than the comparison group ($t = 3.79, df = 250, p = .001$). There were no significant differences in power in the two groups ($t = .44, df = 250, p = .33$) (D. Smith, 1991, 1995).

DR. BARRETT: I see contrasting views of power ranging from the traditional views being more oppressive and moving toward greater autonomy in the feminist view and freedom characterizing the nursing Rogerian view. I have elaborated these different conceptions of power. (See Table 3.1.) It is acausality that allows for freedom in the Rogerian system. Note that these views do not exist on a continuum.

I see nurses as well as clients and others caught in the winds of the shifting paradigms. They are oppressed by the more traditional views of power endorsed not only by bureaucratic institutions of the work place but generally endorsed by other social institutions often beginning with the family, church, school, and the newer views of empowerment and an even more radically autonomous view of power as the capacity to participate knowingly in the nature of change. The latter view maintains that power cannot be given to anyone and that empowerment may mean others decide what we "should" value and be liberated from. Thus, this empowerment type of liberation may also be oppressive and we must guard against rescuing behaviors. The Barrett view of power recognizes reality as a *mutual* process of people *and* their environments. The goal of nurses is power enhancement through changing the environmental pattern. The Rogerian power

Table 3.1   Contrasting Views of Power*

Social Science Traditional Models	Feminist Empowerment Models	Nursing Power Enhancement Model (Barrett, 1990)
Change Causal Determinism	Change Causal	Change Acausal Free will Knowing participation
Power over Oppression Control Domination Force	Power sharing Trust Authority Autonomy	Awareness Choices Freedom to act intentionally Involvement in creating changes
Hierarchical	Liberation	Openness
Separateness	Separateness/ connectedness	Mutual process inseparability
Particulate Mechanistic Reductionistic	Holistic	Unitary
Predetermined outcomes	Desired outcomes	No attachment to outcomes
Predictability	Probability	Unpredictability

*E.A.M. Barrett, © copyright 1993.

theory reflects a new worldview and is antithetical to old worldviews that see power as a causal process and product, that is, as the ability to cause or prevent change. In the traditional view of power, no one is giving it away; power must be taken. In the feminist view, power is shared through empowerment. In the Rogerian view, people have access to their own power that can be enhanced through mutual process with the environment.

3. **Cynthia, based on findings of your study of nurse executives, could it be that you found that power and feminism were not significantly related since the Rogerian view of power is theoretically proposed as being gender free and most studies have shown that there are no significant differences between men and women?**

DR. CAROSELLI: I (Caroselli, 1991) looked at the relationship between power and feminism in 89 female nurse executives in acute care hospitals. The nurse executive is in a pivotal position to influence the delivery of healthcare, since that individual represents the largest

constituency of professional caregivers. The nurse executive, therefore, has a broad arena in which to exercise power and choice. Power
has been viewed in a number of ways, generally from an old world paradigm that emphasizes domination, submission, and control. However,
the theoretical perspective for this study was the Barrettian power theory, which emphasizes awareness, choices, freedom to act intentionally, and involvement in creating change. These concepts are
congruent with much of feminist ideology which seeks to amplify
women's choices. Feminism is an important topic of concern since
most nurse executives, like most nurses, are women, and as such, have
been subjected to stereotypical conditioning relative to women's roles.

Feminism was defined as the promotion of autonomy and equality
for all people, and the abolition of sex role stereotypes. It was measured by the Index of Sex Role Orientation. In response to the question, the Barrettian approach can certainly be seen as transcending the
idea of feminism, so that may have contributed to the lack of support
for the main hypothesis that power and feminism were positively related. A tool to measure feminism from a Rogerian perspective would
be very helpful in elucidating this issue.

Practice Issues

DR. BARRETT: **4. Must one come to know the power theory through
education or is there tacit knowledge of power as knowing participation?**

DR. A. S. SMITH: Let me offer an insight. If practice is Rogerian science-
based, then knowing the theory is prerequisite to its use in practice although there is a theory-practice dialectic.

DR. BARRETT: I agree completely with what you just said and yet, I believe there are people and not only nurses who know the theory without having studied it; they have a tacit knowledge of this view of power
and they also apply it. Yet, we are talking now about the use of the
power theory after it has been learned. In fact, I believe that those who
use the theory in a highly successfully way, actually live the theory.
These role models of power are powerful in ever more diverse ways
when they are free to choose with awareness how they will participate
in changes they wish to create.

DR. BARRETT: **5. Now, another question. In nursing science-based
practice, research utilization is essential. What are the practice
applications pertaining to the administrators, the caregivers,
and the clients regarding power that you have identified from
your research studies?**

DR. CAROSELLI: There are several implications from my study. Departments of nursing face tremendous pressures in this time of cost containment. There is pressure to do more with less, and the drive for increased productivity has become a virtual religion. To achieve greater productivity, every member of the department must have an investment, or sense of ownership, in the mission and goal.

Redesign of the nursing department from a Rogerian/Barrettian perspective can facilitate this sense of ownership in the organization. This ownership may be manifested in greater productivity and possibly better patient "outcomes." This application of the theory "pushes the envelope" toward enhanced operational practicality.

DR. BARRETT: **6. Why are "empowerment" and "personal power" inconsistent with Rogers' science?**

Rogerians are concerned with linguistics. In order to do what you are suggesting, Cynthia requires accuracy and precision in the use of language. Rogers taught us that the Science of Unitary Human Beings like all sciences requires a language of specificity. It requires that whatever ideas are under discussion, consistency with the framework is essential. Webster's Dictionary (1990) defines "empower" as giving official authority, or legal power to. "Em" derives from "en" and means "in." So empowerment means to put power into someone. The notion of empowerment derives from old worldviews and implies a hierarchical position whereby the care "giver" is superior to clients "receiving" the power that caregivers give to them or share with them. Empowerment derives from closed system, causal frameworks. Often such frameworks employ the zero-sum game idea where there is only so much power to go around and the more *you* have, the less *I* have and vice versa. Empowerment implies that as a benevolent patriarchal protector, I as caregiver will empower you so that you can be more powerful, like me. In the Rogerian open systems power theory, clients have power which they can optimize. In deliberative mutual patterning, the nurse facilitates the client's own power enhancement through health patterning. In other words, we promote well-being by assisting people with their knowing participation in change; that is health patterning. Table 3.1 illuminates some of these ideas.

DR. CAROSELLI: This idea is particularly relevant to nursing administration. The nurse executive needs to operate from the idea that power is a characteristic of all unitary human beings. The nurse executive who "empowers" may be nothing more than a lady bountiful bestowing gifts. The problem with such gifts is that they may not be asked for nor wanted, and thus may be less than useful. Therefore, if we truly believe that power is available to all, the notion of a nurse executive endowing a staff member with power is completely inconsistent with the theory. The nurse executive needs to start with the idea that the staff nurse already has access to power.

DR. A. S. SMITH: Frequently, when I describe my study and its findings, people say, "Oh, it's empowerment." But in my reading of the empowerment literature, I find it is mostly atheoretical and focused on groups or communities rather than on the individual.

DR. BARRETT: The term "personal power" is also inappropriate, since it implies separateness and integrality tells us that change occurs in a mutual process and that the human and the environmental energy fields while different by definition are nonetheless inseparable. As long as we focus on power from the 3-D hierarchical closed-system view of the world, power as mutual process will not be perceived. Researchers need to begin to look at power from the perspective of both the human *and* environmental fields in *mutual process.*

DR. BARRETT: **7. What other research-based ideas of power speak to our work with clients?**

DR. A. S. SMITH: I would like to add the idea of patients as partners. In my study, patients who had an active dialogue with their physician asserted their preferences. They negotiated with physicians to postpone invasive events until they had a chance to talk with their families and feel "ready" for the experience. It was really important to them to have time to "think it over."

DR. D. W. SMITH: Research-based practice applications of the power theory include promoting awareness through active listening and the sharing of information, encouraging people to become partners with the healthcare professionals of their choice, and helping people realize that they have power to choose how to respond to events in their lives. Examples in my practice include facilitating a post-polio support group and co-chairing an annual polio survivors' conference in which people hear from health professionals about the topics of their choice and network with them and with one another. On an individual basis, I am guided by the theory in providing people with information, validation, and support. I have also published articles for consumers that were based on the theory of power as mutual process, teaching people how to enhance their power. I am conducting a pilot study on manifestations of power in people giving and receiving Therapeutic Touch. I am hypothesizing a positive relationship between the mutual patterning of human energy and power, spirituality, and symptom relief.

DR. BARRETT: Findings with clients in my private practice support that notion as well as power, optimism, and hope being related. I use the power tool in pattern appraisal incorporating Cowling's (1990) template of experiences, perceptions, and expressions. Butcher (1994) also builds this into his Rogerian research methodology. In my practice, clients who are negative, angry, or pessimistic often score much lower on the power tool. Their hopelessness about life is reflected in the way they live their meager power. They don't feel free to make a difference in their life through initiating changes. They often make unaware choices that have little potential for accelerating changes that they see as desirable but beyond their reach and so they don't reach for options that actually are open to them. They unnecessarily limit their opportunities for creating the changes they desire in their lives.

DR. D. W. SMITH: Examples from the polio survivors in my study that validate that notion were comments such as "Polio is the worst thing that ever happened to me and I would not wish it on any other person." Another person noted very real losses, "A life can't help but be changed by polio. . . . What about not being able to have sex except on your back or in a wheelchair? How about the unending grieving at loss of function—singing, playing catch, walking your baby?"

"Picture . . . a child/girl/woman . . . with one wasted leg, wearing shoes with no heels on them. Consider the effect of this person's appearance, although she has a 165 I.Q., upon entering the plush office of the interviewer for a position commensurate with her abilities. I think you can then understand my jaundiced view of society and humanity. . . ."

At the other end of the spectrum, many examples of power were given. People said things like: "My having had polio has helped me to value life more and to focus on what is really worthwhile and what is not valuable when making choices in life." Another person commented: "Because of insurance problems and local medical professionals' ignorance of possible late effects of polio, I felt compelled to learn more on my own. An unexpected benefit was a feeling of self-'empowerment'."

DR. CAROSELLI: **8. Let me shift this discussion a bit. As we speak, the country is evolving through various models of healthcare reform. Are discussions of conceptual models and, specifically, this power theory topics we no longer have time for?**

DR. A. S. SMITH: Being in nursing service, I'd like to respond. I recently had an opportunity to present my research findings to the advance practice nurses at Detroit Receiving Hospital. They were very interested in possibilities of looking at some of their patternings with patients with the theory in mind. The power concepts made sense to them. One of the staff indicated she knew some folks who made choices before they experienced awareness. This reinforces Barrett's indication that these dimensions are not sequential!

DR. CAROSELLI: The power theory is a practical guide to nurses as they encourage clients to make free and aware choices concerning their health. This is just as relevant for nurses and nursing as it is for clients. For instance, the theory provides a useful framework for career development. The nurse who understands that he/she has power will not wait for opportunity to strike, but will develop the knowledge necessary to make aware choices so that freedom to participate in a career is enhanced. Similarly, the power theory has relevance for political actions by and for nursing. Finally, the power theory can guide research into patient "outcomes," an area that has become particularly persuasive to legislators and third-party payors. While it may seem incongruous to consider theory development in the same breath as reimbursement issues, it is clear that the future of nursing and healthcare is inextricably tied to questions of legislation and reimbursement. Approaching these questions from a nursing science perspective is useful in maintaining a uniquely nursing focus for priority setting.

DR. BARRETT: Rogers gave us many examples when she taught us that theory is often very practical. In the midst of healthcare reform, nursing frameworks such as the Science of Unitary Human Beings will keep the nursing boat from sinking and assure that nursing will not only survive the storm but will survive in a way that the betterment of people will bear a nursing imprimatur. We have the power to see to it!

Methodological Issues, Insights, and Ideas

DR. BARRETT: Several methodological questions have emerged from the research.

9. Can the Power as Knowing Participation in Change Tool (PKPCT) adequately measure differences in power (when they exist) *within* members of a single group?

DR. D. W. SMITH: At this point in its develop, PKPCT scores can be interpreted only as representing greater or lesser power among individuals. PKPCT means for some of the various studies have ranged from a low of 4.9 to a high of 6.0 with a grand mean approximating 5.5. In all of these particular studies a mean of four on the seven-point scale, which would theoretically represent a neutral position, exceeded one standard deviation from the group mean. The consistently high PKPCT means raise questions about the level of discrimination afforded by the instrument. Norms for the PKPCT need to be identified to help address this concern and assist future researchers in interpreting their findings.

DR. BARRETT: **10. Can the PKPCT differentiate *between* different groups?**

There have been relatively few studies comparing different groups. Some have found differences and some have not. Quantitative researchers that have found significant differences including the following: Wynd (1989); Matas Rapacz (1991); Bramlett and Gueldner (1993); Roznowski, (1995); Malinski (1997); Winstead-Fry et al. (1996). In addition, Murray (1989) and Hobbs (1991) used the PKPCT to assign participants to groups designated as powerful and not powerful. Both then did qualitative studies to compare differences in power in the two groups. Each reported that findings validated the quantitative differentiation of power.

DR. D. W. SMITH: In my (D. Smith, 1992) study, neither the PKPCT used as a total measure, nor any of the subscales discriminated between polio survivors and people who had not had polio. Considering Matas Rapacz's findings, my results were curious, since the majority reported having post-polio syndrome, in which pain is a major symptom. I recommend conducting construct validity studies on the PKPCT comparing people judged by a panel of experts to manifest greater power with people judged to manifest lesser power to ascertain when and if researchers can expect the measurement instrument to differentiate among individuals and groups.

DR. BARRETT: Now having heard that the tool differentiated between some groups and not others, let us ponder another question.

11. From a theoretical perspective, should we expect to find differences *between* some groups but not others? In comparing groups, are we asking the right questions? Are there theoretical reasons that suggest no significant difference between some groups? You see, coming from the perspective of the power theory, I'm not convinced that one would expect, for example, polio survivors to score higher than non-polio survivors. In retrospect, how do you see this, Dorothy?

DR. D. W. SMITH: While it is possible that the absence of a significant relationship between power and any aspect of the polio experience indicates that people do not manifest either greater or lesser power associated with polio, the participants' comments suggest that it is more likely that some individuals experience greater power and others experience lesser power associated with polio-related changes. Polio survivors, who manifested the same power as people who have not had polio or any similar illness, may have had greater awareness of themselves as involved in change, therefore greater power, at the time of their acute illness, or greater power during rehabilitation, associated with the will to live or the determination to walk again. It may also be that manifestations of power were less during the acute illness and/or during rehabilitation. To date there have been no studies which indicate whether power is different in an individual when a critical life event is taking place than at times when change is less apparent.

DR. A. S. SMITH: In order to measure the impact of a critical life event on change in power, for example, with patients experiencing coronary artery bypass surgery, we could measure power preoperatively then postoperatively and compare the differences for those who participated in a structured cardiac rehabilitation program and those who elected to do it on their own.

DR. CAROSELLI: It would be very interesting to look at this from an administrative perspective. For instance, many hospitals are altering the skill mix by altering the percentage of RNs to assistive personnel. Many people experience this as a critical event in their professional lives. It would be interesting to compare perceptions of power in nurse executives and staff nurses, before and after this skill mix takes place.

DR. BARRETT: It seems to me that the research findings suggest that we need to test hypotheses that certain health conditions such as chronic pain or crisis or severe distress or the acute phase of illness provide contexts whereby power changes.

12. Cynthia, do you think that the difference in the means of nurse executives of 6.0 in your study (Caroselli, 1991) and the means of staff nurses of 5.5 in Trangenstein's (1988) study suggest that staff nurses have lower power and nurse executives have higher power?

DR. CAROSELLI: As you've stated (Barrett, 1983), power varies in intensity, frequency, and form, and variations in how staff nurses and nurse executives perceive power may reflect variations in the culture of each institution. For instance, an organization that subscribes to a belief of power as knowing participation may manifest this through shared governance, participatory management or some similar model, and may share information much more readily than an organization characterized by a patriarchal approach to management that may be seen as a culture of secrecy. Thus, power as knowing participation may vary among those "in the know" as opposed to those not "in the know."

DR. BARRETT: I would also offer for consideration the idea that there are theoretical reasons that suggest a positive but not statistically significant relationship among some variables and power.

DR. A. S. SMITH: I've been hearing issues defined but I haven't heard much about the strengths of the tool. If I were unfamiliar with the power tool, I might have formulated a jaundiced view of the PKPCT from this discussion we've been having. Perhaps we could briefly summarize some strengths of the tool that have been demonstrated through the research. I'll begin by saying that the tool is useful for ages ranging from adolescence to the oldest old, given they have achieved the reading comprehension level required by the language in the instrument. The tool also works equally well in measuring power in women and men. Consistent with the theory that proposes there are no differences in power between men and women, findings have supported this view. And it has broad applicability in terms of types of populations that can be measured.

Dr. Barrett: **13. How would you summarize the research findings regarding reliability and validity of the PKPCT?**

Dr. D. W. Smith: The tool has consistently been shown to be reliable and valid. This is a major strength of both versions of the PKPCT. (See Table 3.2.) Factor Loadings $\geq .40$ indicate construct validity. Factor loadings ranged from .56 to .70 in Barrett's (1983) study.

Dr. Barrett: Cynthia and I (Barrett & Caroselli, 1996) have written an article on methodological issues of the PKPCT where we discuss in addition to instrument sensitivity, issues of social desirability, response set, complexity of language, clarity of directions, use of the retest items as measures of acquiescence, and other psychometric considerations.

SUMMARY

Dr. Barrett: Perhaps we can summarize by means of four final questions posed to the reader as a starting point for further inquiry.

14. **First, from the theoretical standpoint, "What is the significance of power as participating knowingly for a person's health?"**

15. **Second, in terms of methodology, how can both qualitative and quantitative studies help us understand the relationship between power and health?**

16. **Third, what are the practice implications of the significance of power for a person's health?**

17. **Finally, how can health patterning modalities such as imagery, Therapeutic Touch, meditation, humor, relaxation, use of color, sound, motion, and light facilitate movement from the theoretical to the practice arena where the Science of Unitary Human Beings provides the guiding scientific light?**

Table 3.2 Estimates of Reliability for the Power as Knowing Participation in Change Tool (PKPCT)

	PKPCT, Version I				PKPCT, Version II					
	Barrett 1983* N = 625	D. Smith 1991	Malinski 1995 N = 400	Barrett 1996 N = 586	Trangenstein 1988 N = 326	Wynd 1989 N = 106	Bramlett 1990 N = 81	Rizzo 1990 N = 84	Caroselli 1991 N = 89	Barrett 1996 N = 586
Awareness	.63	.88	.89	.91	.86	.86	.82	.87	.83	.89
Choices	.75	.89	.90	.91	.88	.90	.81	.81	.87	.91
Freedom to act intentionally	.95	.93	.91	.92	.89	.91	.82	.87	.85	.92
Involvement in creating changes	.99	.93	.92	.93	.92	.92	.84	.87	.89	.93
Total		.97	.97	.97	.96			.94	.95	.97

*Variance of factor scores used as estimate of reliability. All other reliabilities were computed using Cronbach's alpha.

We propose that the completed work on power can serve as a magnet to bring new energy and ideas together to create future discoveries of power as knowing participation in change.

REFERENCES

Barrett, E. A. M. (1983). *An empirical investigation of Martha E. Rogers' principle of helicy: The relationship between human field motion and power.* Unpublished doctoral dissertation, New York University, New York. (University Microfilms No. 84-06278).

Barrett, E. A. M. (1986). The principle of helicy: The relationship of human field motion and power. In V. M. Malinski (Ed.), *Explorations on Martha Rogers' science of unitary human beings* (pp. 173–188). Norwalk, CT: Appleton-Century-Crofts.

Barrett, E. A. M. (1989). A nursing theory of power for nursing practice: Derivation from Rogers' paradigm. In J. Riehl-Sisca (Ed.), *Conceptual models for nursing practice* (3rd ed., pp. 207–217). Norwalk, CT: Appleton & Lange.

Barrett, E. A. M. (1990a). An instrument to measure power as knowing participation in change. In O. Strickland & C. Waltz (Eds.), *The measurement of nursing outcomes: Measuring client self-care and coping skills* (Vol. 4, pp. 159–180). New York: Springer.

Barrett, E. A. M. (1990b). Health patterning with clients in a private practice environment. In E. A. M. Barrett (Ed.), *Visions of Rogers' science-based nursing* (pp. 105–115). New York: NLN Press.

Barrett, E. A. M. (1996). *The relationship of human field motion and power: A replication and extension.* Manuscript in preparation.

Barrett, E. A. M., & Caroselli, C. (1996). *Methodological issues and insights related to the power as knowing participation in change instrument.* Manuscript submitted for publication.

Bramlett, M. (1990). *The relationship of creativity, power, and reminiscence in the elderly.* Unpublished doctoral dissertation, Medical College of Georgia, Athens.

Bramlett, M., & Gueldner, S. H. (1993). Reminiscence: A viable option to enhance power in elders. *Clinical Nurse Specialist, 7*(2), 68–74.

Butcher, H. (1994). *A unitary field pattern portrait of dispiritedness in later life.* Unpublished doctoral dissertation, University of South Carolina, Columbia.

Caroselli, C. (1991). *The relationship of power and feminism in women nurse executives in acute care hospitals.* Unpublished doctoral dissertation, New York University, New York.

Cowling, W. R. (1990). A template for unitary pattern-based nursing practice. In E. A. M. Barrett (Ed.), *Visions of Rogers' science-based nursing* (pp. 45–65). New York: NLN Press.

Hobbs, M. B. (1991). *Manifestations influencing empowerment in the educational environment of baccalaureate nursing students.* Unpublished doctoral dissertation, University of Alabama, Birmingham.

Malinski, V. (1997). The relationship of temporal experience and power as knowing participation in change in depressed and non-depressed women. *Patterns of Rogerian knowing.* New York: NLN Press.

Matas Rapacz, K. (1991). *Human patterning and chronic pain.* Unpublished doctoral dissertation, Case Western Reserve University, Cleveland, OH.

Murray, L. (1989). *An exploration of the factors of empowerment as perceived by persons with end stage renal failure.* Unpublished doctoral dissertation, University of Alabama, Birmingham.

Nunnally, J. C. (1978). *Psychometric theory* (2nd ed.). New York: McGraw-Hill.

Phillips, J. R. (1990). Changing human potentials and future visions of nursing: A human field image perspective. In E. A. M. Barrett (Ed.), *Visions of Rogers' science-based nursing* (pp. 13–25). New York: NLN Press.

Rizzo, J. (1990). *The relationship of life satisfaction, purpose in life, and power in older adults.* Unpublished doctoral dissertation, New York University, New York.

Rogers, M. E. (1970). *An introduction to the theoretical basis of nursing.* Philadelphia: F. A. Davis.

Rogers, M. E. (1990). Nursing: Science of unitary, irreducible human beings: Update, 1990. In E. A. M. Barrett (Ed.), *Visions of Rogers' science-based nursing* (pp. 5–11). New York: NLN Press.

Roznowski, H. (1995). *Diabetes education: Knowledge, power, and change.* Unpublished master's thesis, Northern Michigan University.

Silva, M. C., & Sorrell, J. M. (1992). Testing of nursing theory: Critique and philosophical expansion. *Advances in Nursing Science, 14*(4), 12–23.

Smith, A. S. (1993). *Discovering patients' perceptions of participation in managing chronic illness.* Unpublished doctoral dissertation, Wayne State University, Detroit, MI.

Smith, A. S. (1995). Patient participation in changing behaviors, *Home Healthcare Nurse, 13*(2), 45–49.

Smith, D. W. (1991). *A study of power and spirituality in polio survivors using the nursing model of Martha E. Rogers.* Unpublished doctoral dissertation, New York University, New York.

Smith, D. W. (1995). Power and spirituality in polio survivors: A study based on Rogers' science. *Nursing Science Quarterly, 8,* 133–139.

Trangenstein, P. A. (1988). *Relationships of power and job diversity to job satisfaction and job involvement: An empirical investigation of Rogers' principle of integrality.* Unpublished doctoral dissertation, New York University, New York.

Winstead-Fry, P., Paletta, J., Barrett, E. A. M., Krause, K., Lee, W. H., Nojima, Y., & Olson, H. (1996). *International study of Rogers' conceptual model.* Manuscript submitted for publication.

Wynd, C. A. (1989). *The use of guided imagery to enhance power for smoking behavior change.* Unpublished doctoral dissertation, Case Western Reserve University, Cleveland, OH.

4

Unitary Perspectives on Methodological Practices

Elizabeth Ann Manhart Barrett, W. Richard Cowling III, Judith Treschuk Carboni, and Howard K. Butcher

*T*he Science of Unitary Human Beings (Rogers, 1992) expresses an onto-logical view that creates theoretical excitement and methodological chal-lenge. The evolution of unitary theoretical thinking has been accompanied by methodological pondering and searching to respond to the knowledge development needs of the discipline of nursing. Underlying the scholarly debates about methods in the public arena of conferences and journals are individual stories of researchers seeking the methodological practices that serve an alternative unitary world view for nursing. In this chapter, we de-scribe the methodological journeys of four scholars who developed pro-grams of research grounded in the Science of Unitary Human Beings. These journeys are shared to enlighten and encourage those who seek answers to the methodological challenges of unitary science.

THE CASE FOR CONTINUING USE OF QUANTITATIVE METHODS IN ROGERIAN PATTERNS OF INQUIRY

Elizabeth Ann Manhart Barrett

Long ago and far away I had a dream. The dream began to come true when in 1970 I became a registered nurse at age 35. Three years later, I had an epiphany! This awakening came one Spring Friday afternoon as I began reading Rogers' (1970) *An Introduction to the Theoretical Basis of Nursing;* an all-at-once tacit knowing that somehow Rogers' work would play a key role in actualizing my dream during the rest of my career.

Once upon another time, just three years later, I began living a wondrous waking dream, having chosen to move from Indiana to New York to study Rogers' work as the substantive knowledge for the PhD degree. Ten years earlier I would have never predicted any of this in my wildest dreams. Yet, this is the unpredictable way the universe works! There I was, living across the street from the hallowed halls where Rogers taught "Science of Man" (in those days many still described humankind this way). I was truly stunned when I discovered that she would actually be my teacher—and for an entire year. This was only the first of many surprises about the accessibility of this remarkable woman whom I had mistakenly visioned as isolated in an ivory tower. Instead, she came to class pushing a shopping cart full of handouts!

Meanwhile, I was beginning to hear many voices echoing "yes, but." YES, Rogers' work is interesting, important, and she has made significant contributions to nursing. BUT, you cannot use Rogers' framework as a basis for research, since "it" cannot be measured. Notice that the question at that time, "Can 'it' be measured?" is very different from the current question, "Is it appropriate to measure 'it'"?

Then a minor miracle occurred, serendipitously as many miracles do. After two years of reading, searching, and attempting to describe power within Rogers' conceptual system, as it was known at that time, I was attending the 1978 Nurse Theorist Conference, a truly historic event. The excitement was intense. Rogers was speaking on stage, about to say something I had heard her say many times in class; yet, this time it was different. Suddenly when I heard her say "Human beings can knowingly participate in change," the light bulb went on! At that moment, I made the connection that power, a concept not then addressed in Rogers' science, is essentially knowing participation in change. Ah-ha! That's it! Eureka!

The struggle to define and describe a Rogerian view of power began. Everywhere, everyone seemed to be saying, "But how will you measure it?" Indeed, the few instruments available to measure power reflected old worldviews. I would need to develop an instrument to operationalize power.

In the late 1970s at New York University, quantitative methodology was dominant. Placing the event in space time is crucial to understanding not only the thrust of my work but the work of all the Rogerian researchers who came before and after me. While doctoral students had previously investigated constructs considered relevant to understanding unitary persons and their environments, it was not until 1977 when Rawnsley framed her study solely within the Science of Unitary Human Beings (SUHB) that hypotheses were derived from this framework (Ference, 1986).

Meanwhile, there were several of us in the nursing doctoral program at NYU who were striving to break this new ground and our camaraderie was intellectually stimulating and mutually supportive. We were on a quest to demonstrate that theorems derived from Rogers' framework could be measured. This search for ways to operationalize abstract Rogerian conceptualizations was our mission, our passion, and our commitment.

Eventually my ideas began to take shape. I was simultaneously developing the power theory along with a semantic differential approach to measuring power. After many meetings with Dr. Rogers, by now a member of my dissertation committee, she finally said, "Now I see what you've been trying to get at all along. You just might have something there." The rest of my power story is history, as evidenced by my publications.

Since the early 1980s, research-based knowledge in the SUHB has been accumulating at an accelerating pace through use of an array of traditional and new methods (Caroselli & Barrett, 1996; Dykeman & Loukissa, 1993). The story of yesterday is not the story of today nor will it be the story of tomorrow.

My process is open-ended, like science itself. I can only tell you where I am now; the future is unpredictable although it is a delight to contemplate. These are times of tremendous excitement and great adventure. I go forth each day to participate knowingly in creating my reality, hoping somehow, some way to give back through my teaching, research, and practice some of the many gifts I have received in my life and my work. I hope this brief glimpse of my emerging journey will encourage others to follow their dreams. And my dream goes on.

Advocating use of both qualitative and quantitative research approaches is a position I have long maintained. The arguments do not need to be repeated here, only updated. In 1990, I urged the pursuit of a unique Rogerian research methodology. Since then we have witnessed the birth of three new qualitative approaches. Are they unique Rogerian research methodologies? There can be no doubt the methods created by Butcher, Carboni, and Cowling are moving us along in exciting ways.

Currently, the methods debate has begun to focus on the issue of whether or not Rogerian researchers should discard quantitative methods altogether. What is to be gained by limiting our perspective? Why select "either/or" when we can have "and"? At this time I don't believe the evidence is convincing enough to discard quantitative methodology; it has proved useful to Rogerian science and other new worldview sciences such as modern physics.

"Research methods are not paradigm specific but should be selected on the basis of whether they fit with the purposes of an investigation" (Ford-Gilboe, Campbell, & Berman, 1995, p. 14). In quantitative endeavors, despite use of statistical methods, the conceptualization of the problem is not required to be in sync with the positivist paradigm (Goswami, 1993). While the famous research dictum, "Correlation does not mean causation" speaks well for Rogers' acausal system, Pedhazur (1982) follows this with additional comment, "Nor does any other index prove causation, regardless of whether the index was derived from data collected in experimental or in nonexperimental research" (p. 579).

While use of quantitative methods may present a measurement paradox in juxtaposition to the ontology and epistemology of the SUHB, an argument has been presented here and elsewhere for keeping both the quantitative and qualitative doors wide open. While acknowledging the incongruence of linear and reductionistic formulas with the Rogerian worldview, quantitative methodology allows hypotheses derived from theories to be tested with a specificity unique to numerical approaches. From this perspective, methods are viewed as tools of science and are not to be confused with the science itself. To illustrate, consider that one would not confuse the computer with the information that it stores and uses. The critical ontological and epistemological congruence is reflected in the nature of the questions asked and their theoretical conceptualization.

Rogers (1988) reminded us that there can be no final words or ultimate proclamations.

Nevertheless, her position on the methods debate is quite clear (1992, 1994a, 1994b), "There are many arguments about qualitative and quantitative methods. . . . I have heard people say that quantitative methods would not work in Rogerian science. That is not true" (Rogers, 1994a, p. 8). For now, I rest my case.

CASE STUDY: A PATTERN APPRECIATION METHOD

W. Richard Cowling III

Since my New York University days, days of immersion in the Science of Unitary Human Beings, I have wandered through the vast land of academic research and scholarship taking many divergent paths. Recently, I realized that all these wanderings were beneficial and I am more convinced than ever of the need for advanced methods that address the theoretical perspectives posed within the Science of Unitary Human Beings. I have written about the process of doing science from a unitary perspective using more traditional methods and more recently have advocated for a new methodological perspective for practice and research that involves a process called unitary pattern appreciation. The case method approach places the unitary pattern appreciation process within an implementation framework for doing science.

I started out as a true unitary nonbeliever, in spite of master's content on the framework and attendance at a national presentation by Dr. Rogers. An enduring attraction, that at one time I described as intellectual, occurred in the summer of 1979 while listening to Martha lecture at New York University. This attraction to this view of human beings is the abiding theme that has lived through my academic and professional career. Without understanding this attraction, it is difficult to understand the methodological choices to which I have been led.

The view of reality espoused by Rogers is one of humans as patterning energy fields evolving in simultaneous mutual process with environmental energy fields in a pandimensional universe growing and changing unpredictably. without causal connectivity. It is a view that reconceptualized humans beyond physical, psychological, and spiritual as unitary entities implying a unity of substance or existence that releases the scientist and practitioner from any notion of parts. Later, I came to realize that this also meant that what appears to us as "part" is really manifestation of pattern; everything we encounter reflects unitary existence because in a world of unitary being, parts simply do not exist. In addition, four dimensionality, later to become pandimensionality, took me beyond all the old concepts of space and time as bounded and linear respectively. Finally, while I was first challenged by the idea of unpredictability and acausality (why would we participate if we cannot change things?), I came to appreciate that these conceptualizations offered a wide universe of opportunity for change beyond any constraints.

All this meant that I was forced to see what I had experienced and known in clinical practice differently. The unitary nature of human beings helped me begin to understand why despite blatant physical or emotional scars, individual patients seemed to display a wholeness that transcended the particular damage. Likewise, some individuals with seemingly minor limitations experienced a deeper pain that was larger than any particular small aspect of physical alteration or emotional disturbance. In other words, what was apparent on the surface belied a deeper patterning of unitary existence. It became increasingly more relevant that the surface display of information be considered in the context of unitary patterning and that pattern be given attention as the referent for practice and for creating a knowledge base of science for the practice of nursing.

Pandimensionality and the integral nature of human-environmental energy field pattern led me to understand that human beings carry collapsed space-time experience and their environment around with them as relative presence. A mother experiences her child at a distance. What is past pain is not past at all, but feels like it is happening now. Love, despair, and struggle do not have immediate environmental referents always. What may happen in the future is experienced as immediate. These realizations of pandimensionality and integrality of human-environmental energy, provide a context for opening nurses to clients' experiences in new ways.

The acausal nature of change also meant that there was a shift away from intervention for the sake of specific outcomes to a participation with people for the sake of deeper knowing, what I have called unitary knowing, and an opening to a universe of possibilities for change (unpredictability). This is a shared knowing that unfolds into actions. I liken this process to the metaphor of "dawn"; it dawned on me that the most important thing I could do at this moment is change that behavior. This means that actions flow from realizations or "dawnings" upon participants. In this conceptual model change is inevitable, but there is choice for knowing participation in natural change. This also means that form is less significant than experience.

More and more I became aware that the conceptualizations of this unitary perspective would mean offering alternatives to our previous understandings of human health-illness. The next aspect of my journey was the dawning realization of what it would mean to have a scientific foundation for practice based on these unitary conceptualizations.

My dissertation was a theory testing, descriptive, correlational study of correlates of unitary patterning. The results of this research yielded support for the hypothesized relationship, struggle to get the findings published finally in a psychology journal, and uneasiness about the meaning of what I had done. I spent a number of years doing and seeking to do research hiding my conceptual yearnings and using traditional approaches to research and knowledge development. I was convinced by others that if I got a mainstream research program launched, later I could do what I really wanted. At the same time I became heavily involved with teaching doctoral courses and working with doctoral students. Much of what I taught was about the congruence of worldviews or conceptual systems, theories, philosophies of science, and methods. I learned and taught about discovered and emerging qualitative and constructivist modes of inquiry for developing nursing science.

It was like living in two worlds, trying to launch fundable research projects, and knowing passionately that what mattered most was launching a program of research in the Science of Unitary Human Beings. Admittedly, I was able to write theoretical and practice-based articles and chapters on unitary science and I was able to conduct a practice in which I attempted to integrate the unitary perspective. However, this was so superfluous to my major work that I describe this experience to many doctoral students and colleagues as running around a huge pool of inviting water teaching others to swim . . . never swimming myself, always directing, describing in great detail the nature of the water and the requisites for swimming well . . . and I was good at it . . . all the while never getting wet. Lately, I have begun to wade and actually take some strokes. Discovering and realizing pattern appreciation in the context of case method meant it was time to dive.

The unitary pattern appreciation case method evolved out of the creation of a template and later guiding assumptions for unitary practice and research. Pattern appreciation is a central aspect of guiding assumptions for unitary practice and research and is more fully explicated elsewhere in this text. Pattern appreciation is a way of approaching and deepening one's understanding of pattern. The process of pattern appreciation involves being aware of, sensitive to, and grateful for the uniqueness of another's pattern. Pattern appreciation is conscious evolution in my thinking from appraisal or assessment. Pattern appreciation is approached through opening one's self to the experience, perception, and expressions of another as representative of pattern manifestations. Pattern appreciation requires the researcher/practitioner to embrace an inclusive view of what counts as pattern information including a wide array of phenomena that are often discarded in other theoretical perspectives. Phenomena are considered to be energetic manifestations.

Pattern information is sought through multiple modes of awareness by the nurse researcher/practitioner. Information is configured into a pattern profile based on a process of synopsis and synthesis. Synopsis involves looking at data from experience, perception, and expressions to seek the clearest and fullest picture of unitary pattern that is reflected. Synthesis seeks a coherent set of concepts and principles that cover all the data viewed synoptically. In a case study method approach, this means that the concepts and principles would be relevant to the particular case. Synopsis and synthesis lead to a pattern construction called a pattern profile.

Pattern profiles can be derived or constructed for either research or practice or both depending on the negotiated purpose of the situation that exists between the scientist/practitioner and the person who agrees to participate. Pattern profile is a construction that is shared with the participant for verification. The central question is whether the profile reflects pattern from his or her perspective. The form of the profile varies depending on the individual situation. Appreciation shapes knowledge development and action within the context of the case as it emerges from the process of seeking to know and constructing the profile. Knowledge can take many forms including theoretical and practical.

The design of the pattern appreciation case method evolved from the journey of seeking to create a context for knowledge development from a unitary science perspective and to understand human phenomena relevant to practice through the lens of a unitary worldview. It grew into a scientist/practitioner model of nursing that is congruent with unitary concepts and ideals and consistent with my own attractions to this worldview and passions to live out a life of practice and science that is both unitary and transformative. Swimming requires immersion in and participation with water. Unitary pattern appreciation case method is my swimming in the unitary sea.

THE ART OF CREATING METHOD:
A ROGERIAN PROCESS OF INQUIRY

Judith Treschuk Carboni

Approaching nursing research from a Rogerian perspective has provided an exciting and challenging opportunity to create a new and innovative research methodology grounded in the Science of Unitary Human Beings. Inherent in this effort has been a commitment to logical congruency of philosophy, theory, and method and the unwavering conviction that if we are to do nursing research, then nursing theory must guide the inquiry process. The successful development of a unitary research method encompassed a deep and rich journey into unitary theoretical thinking and earnest pondering of the nature of unitary nursing, the nature of change, and the possibility of qualitative measurement.

The first step in the journey included an exploration of the philosophical and epistemological threads of Rogers' conceptual system (Carboni,

1991). This exploration led to several realizations: unitary nursing practice could not be articulated nor enacted from a linear or causal perspective, thus nursing could not "do" or "intervene"; and, likewise, unitary research based on Rogers' conceptual system could not logically address particularistic conceptualizations or quantitatively testable hypotheses, thus all quantitative methodologies were incongruent. Given these two conclusions, several significant questions arose. If nursing practice was neither linear nor causal, and if nursing did not "intervene," then did one conclude that change did not occur? Being fully committed to nursing practice and the belief that nurses *did* make a difference, the denial of the manifestation of change was impossible. Change did indeed occur, but it was clearly different than the three-dimensional notion of change and could only be understood in terms of the nonlinear and dynamic movement of energy field patterns. The acceptance that change within a unitary reality was possible led to consideration of a second question: if quantitative measurement was incongruent with a unitary reality, did that then mean that Rogers' conceptual system could not be tested and change manifested through Rogerian nursing practice could not be measured? This second question became particularly significant in light of the generally held conviction that qualitative methodologies were inductive and could only result in description and deeper understanding, not in testing or refinement of a priori theory. Given the judgment that all quantitative methodologies were incongruent with a unitary reality and the fact that the prevailing views of qualitative methods excluded the possibility of testing Rogers' Science of Unitary Human Beings or any unitary theories derived from this conceptual system, the challenge was to expand understanding of quantitative methodology and give consideration to the possibility of testing and measuring from a new perspective. Innovative understanding of the nature of unitary change and the possibility of creatively measuring that change became quite feasible when the view for considering these phenomena was altered from a causal, three-dimensional perspective to one that was dynamic, acausal, nonlinear, and timeless. This led to the second step on the pathway to the maturing of a Rogerian process of inquiry.

In this next step, attention was given to the idea of qualitative measurement and the development of instruments to measure unitary constructs (Carboni, 1992). Integral to this exploration was acknowledgment of energy field patterns as the only reliable and valid indicators of the whole. In terms of construct development, this meant that any construct purported to be unitary in nature had to be *inclusive* of the Science of Unitary Human Beings. Of equal significance in this exploration was the affirmation that measurement did not necessarily equate to assigning numbers to particular responses or behaviors that could only be understood empirically. It was proposed that there existed an alternative vision of measurement that was grounded in a different worldview. This second view of measurement, called *creative measurement,* did not rely on the merely empirically knowable, but honored understanding and knowing unbounded reality from multiple sources of experiences, expressions, and perceptions, all of which transcended empirical boundaries. Emergent from this exploration was the development of the unitary construct of the healing human field—environmental field relationship and the instrument entitled Mutual Exploration of the Healing Human Field—Environmental Field Relationship. This instrument was designed to provide qualitative measurement of the manifestation/presence of this unitary phenomenon. This second portion of the journey had revealed that Rogerian research did *not* have to be restricted to description and understanding, but could strive to test and measure unitary constructs/theories derived from Rogers' conceptual system. Furthermore, in order to accomplish this, the Rogerian researcher did not have to resort to incongruent three-dimensional quantitative methodologies, but rather it was possible and theoretically acceptable to measure qualitatively. This was another step closer to the realization of a Rogerian research methodology; however, there remained one more diversion in this admittedly nonlinear journey.

Because Rogers' conceptual system had frequently been identified as too abstract and general and not empirically knowable, numerous Rogerian researchers had mistakenly attempted to develop middle-range theories and constructs in order to test the conceptual system. These middle-range theories and constructs called for placing boundaries on designated aspects of reality and were thus incongruent with Rogers' unbounded, pandimensional worldview. If the critique was correct that most of the Rogerian research done had erred both in the identification of particularistic conceptualizations and in its attempts to measure quantitatively, then how could one successfully conceptualize and measure Rogerian nursing practice and its manifestations of field patterning? The vision was to practice Rogerian nursing and to creatively measure the manifestations of field patterning that emerged during co-participation of the nurse and client in this process. In order for this to happen, a theory of Rogerian nursing practice had to be derived from Rogers' conceptual system and it had to reflect the system in its entirety. This was the beginning of the evolution of a theory of Rogerian nursing practice entitled "Enfolding Health-as-Wholeness-and-Harmony" (Carboni, 1995b). This theory provided an evolutionary understanding of Rogerian nursing practice and provided the conceptual understanding necessary for the identification and testing of theoretical statements.

Having followed the unitary path for so long and with such careful attention to all the theoretical practice and research implications of completely honoring Rogers' conceptual system, it was now time to do some actual research. The groundwork had been laid. It had been demonstrated that it was possible to test the Science of Unitary Human Beings and that this could only be done qualitatively. How one might measure qualitatively had been explored and new instruments to measure unitary constructs had been developed. A unitary theory of Rogerian nursing practice had been derived from the Science of Unitary Human Beings and had made it possible to test the conceptual system in its entirety. All this had been accomplished, but not surprisingly, there existed no extant qualitative research methodology that was congruent with all the tenets of Rogers' Science of Unitary Human Beings, including the possibilities of measuring qualitatively and transcending space and time. Thus, the journey next involved a deep and complete exploration of all the ontological and epistemological assumptions of the Science of Unitary Human Beings and a discussion of the implications they held for the emergence of a creative and original process of inquiry.

A Rogerian process of inquiry congruent with unitary reality emerged from this deep exploration and has been described in depth elsewhere (Carboni, 1995a). It was steadfastly affirmed that Rogerian research could only be done qualitatively and in complete equality with all co-participants of the study. Because of the nature of unitary reality, the focus of any Rogerian study had to be human and environmental energy fields and could only take place within a pandimensional research field where it was neither constrained by the limitations imposed by determinism and causal laws nor bound to time and context. Furthermore, the possibility of testing Rogerian theory through qualitative measurement was presented, along with the impossibility of ever separating deductive data from inductive data. This methodology was presented as transcending the boundaries imposed by time and space and thus allowed for the simultaneous inductive emergence of data *and* the testing of a priori theory.

The Rogerian process of inquiry has emerged from well thought-out, well articulated and coherent philosophical and theoretical positions and informs us that the determination of methodology emerges not from the research question one asks, nor from the complexity of the phenomena being studied, but rather from the worldview on which one's theoretical framework is based. Furthermore, it acknowledges that the question is far more than choosing a particular method; it is a question of the entire process of inquiry one chooses to follow. The potential for refining and deepening Rogers' conceptual system and developing new unitary theory awaits the courageous and inquisitive researcher who is willing to follow this path.

THE ART OF CREATING METHOD

Howard K. Butcher

The creation of new methods for research is a creative artistic endeavor. The art of creating art is like the art of creating science. This story illustrates my creative journey constructing the Unitary Field Pattern Portrait (UFPP) research method (see Figure 4.1).

After completing my master's thesis at the University of Toronto, I decided to pursue doctoral studies with Richard Cowling at University of South Carolina. Initially I planned on building on my master's thesis by investigating the relationship between guided imagery and knowing participation in change. However, concerns about the choice of methodology emerged immediately in my course work based on the new knowledge I was learning through the study of recent advances in philosophy of science. Numerous scholars have asserted that there should be a congruence

Figure 4.1   The Unitary Field Pattern Portrait Research Method

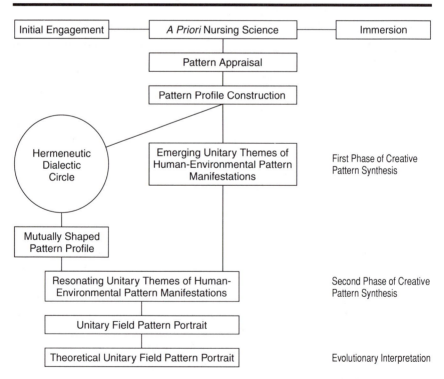

between a paradigm's ontology, epistemology, and methodology. In addition, quantitative designs seemed to have ontological and epistemological assumptions about causality, reductionism, particularism, control, prediction, objectivity, and linearity that are clearly inconsistent with Rogers' unitary worldview. New paradigm science requires the development of new methodologies. An understanding of pandimensional unitary human beings and their environment is best advanced through the generation of new knowledge by methodologies developed to be consistent with the tenets of Rogers' unitary ontology and mutual process epistemology.

Since clues to developing a Rogerian research method are embedded in the epistemological and ontological tenets of Rogerian Science, I used a framework by Morgan (1983) to analyze Rogers' ontology and epistemology (Butcher, 1994a, 1994b). I identified kaleidoscopic patterns and symphony as essential epistemological metaphors embedded in Rogers' epistemology. Each metaphor became a guidepost for developing a "favored methodology." Based on my analysis of Rogers' unitary ontology and mutual process epistemology, the method needed to focus on the appraisal of experiences, perceptions, and expressions as unitary pattern manifestations emerging from the human-environmental energy field mutual process. The researcher and the researched-into are integral and in mutual process with one another and the researcher uses pandimensional modes of awareness to apprehend kaleidoscopic and symphonic pattern manifestations associated with human betterment and well-being.

A key foundation for developing criteria for Rogerian inquiry was Lincoln and Guba's (1985) description of naturalistic inquiry or "constructivist paradigm" (Guba & Lincoln, 1989). The ontology and epistemology of constructivism paralleled the ontology and epistemology of Rogerian science. Both share views of reality as being characterized by: multiple realities, mutual process, continuous change, integrality, openness, indivisible wholes, unpredictability, natural context, increasing diversity, and multiple modes of awareness. With some minor modifications, I was able to illustrate how the constructivist ontology and epistemology were congruent with the ontology and epistemology of Rogerian science (Butcher, 1994b). In addition, Guba and Lincoln (1989) proposed a constructivist research methodology and I reasoned that if the ontology and epistemology of Rogerian science and constructivism were congruent, then the constructivist methodology may shed some light on the development of a Rogerian methodology.

A second foundation for developing the UFPP method was Cowling's template for Unitary Pattern-Based research. Richard's description of the appraisal of experiences, perceptions, and expressions provided the focus and process for apprehending manifestations of human-environmental field patterns using multiple modes of awareness. Richard also described the process of understanding pattern information within a unitary context and developing a pattern profile as a means for describing the person's human-environmental field pattern.

While developing the method, I was able to take a course with Dr. Rosemarie Parse on "Creative Sciencing." Parse described the art of creating science in the same way Stephen Sondheim described the process of creating art in the Broadway musical "Sunday in the Park with George." I had seen the musical in 1985 and often listened to the soundtrack and had a video of the play. I vividly recall how over months of constructing the UFPP method, the lyrics of a song "Putting it Together" from the musical would resonate with me:

> *Bit by bit, Putting it together . . . Piece by piece . . . Only way to make art. Every movement makes a contribution, Every detail plays a part. Having just the vision's no solution, Everything depends on execution. Putting it together is what counts . . . Small amounts, adding up make a work of art, First you need a good foundation, Otherwise it's risky from the start . . . Link by link. Making the connections . . . Art isn't easy . . . Have to hold on to your vision . . . The art of making art, is putting it together, Bit by bit. (Sondheim, 1984)*

While the lyrics seem to describe a linear process, in actuality, the process of "putting it together" was a nonlinear creative process of "flow" (Csikszentmihalyi, 1996). Flow experiences are potentially creative experiences that include concentration, absorption, joy, deep involvement, and a sense of accomplishment (Csikszentmihalyi, 1996). The process of creating the UFPP included intense immersion into the study of Rogers' ontology and epistemology and the question of an appropriate methodology. Awareness and action merged together. Long periods of incubation were imbued with creative insights and punctuated with epiphanies. An epiphany is an ethereal sense of *ah-hah* experiences, a sudden awareness and synthesis of knowledge into grand new pattern (Mitchell, 1996). For example, the moment I read Guba and Lincoln's description of the constructivist paradigm, in a sudden flash, I saw a new synthesis between constructivist inquiry and Cowling's methodology. Constant evaluation allowed me to decide which insights and paths were worth pursuing. In my dreams at night, ideas and insights would appear, and often I got up at 2 or 3 AM and worked another 2 hours composing method on the computer. I avoided distractions and often I totally lost my sense of self, time, and surroundings. As I was deeply immersed in the process of constructing the method, I often lost my sense of time by becoming totally enraptured in a process. My immersion and engagement in constructing the method had its own unique rhythm. Nonlocal synchronicities also were part of the journey. While studying Guba and Lincoln's constructivism, I simultaneously discovered a new book by Capra and Steindl-Rast (1991, p. 123) in which Capra stated "the people who are in the forefront of this [new paradigm science] research tend to say that a school known as 'constructivism' is the appropriate epistemology." Nearly at the same time, I met Judith Carboni at the 4th Rogerian Conference, who to my amazement, also was using Lincoln and Guba's criteria of constructivist inquiry to develop her initial criteria for Rogerian inquiry. Through in-depth study, I elaborated the method components by weaving together the philosophical and epistemological arguments that provided a rationale for each phase and process of the UFPP (Butcher, 1994b).

Csikszentmihalyi (1996) also describes how creative environments are integral to the creative process. In the early 1990s, the University of South Carolina was the "right place" to be for engaging in Rogerian research. There were several Rogerians on faculty and an inspiring environment which nurtured creativity and scholarship was created by Richard Cowling and all my committee members. The program of study also created opportunities for me to consult with Margaret Newman and Rosemarie Parse during the early phases of UFPP development. I was able to take an independent study in Rogerian Science with Sarah Gueldner and Martha Rogers on the beaches of North Carolina. On the beaches, there were opportunities for long dialogues with Martha Rogers and aspiring Rogerian scholars. The beautiful and stimulating surroundings catalyzed the creative process of synthesis.

The first application of the UFPP research method was an investigation into the experience of dispiritedness in later life (Butcher, in press). Maryellen Dye, a doctoral student at the Medical College of South Carolina, plans to use the UFPP to study traumatic injury. Hopefully other Rogerian researchers will find the UFPP useful for advancing Rogerian Science concept and theory development while composing their own stories of creative sciencing.

REFERENCES

Butcher, H. K. (1994a). The unitary field pattern portrait method: Development of research method within Rogers' science of unitary human beings. In M. Madrid & E. A. M. Barrett (Eds.), *Rogers's art of nursing practice.* New York: NLN Press.

Butcher, H. K. (1994b). *A unitary field pattern portrait of dispiritedness in later life.* Doctoral dissertation, University of South Carolina.

Butcher, H. K. (1996). A unitary field pattern portrait of dispiritedness in later life. *Visions: The Journal of Rogerian Nursing Science, 4,* 41–58.

Butcher, H. K. & Parker, N. (1990). Guided imagery within Martha Rogers' science of unitary beings: An experimental study. In E. A. M. Barrett (Ed.), *Visions of Rogers' science-based nursing* (pp. 269–285). New York: NLN Press.

Capra, F., & Steindl-Rast, D. (1991). *Belonging to the universe.* San Francisco: Harper & Row.

Carboni, J. T. (1991). A Rogerian theoretical tapestry. *Nursing Science Quarterly, 4,* 130-136.

Carboni, J. T. (1992). Instrument development and the measurement of unitary constructs. *Nursing Science Quarterly 5,* 134-142.

Carboni, J. T. (1995a). A Rogerian process of inquiry. *Nursing Science Quarterly, 8,* 22-37.

Carboni, J. T. (1995b). Enfolding health-as-wholeness-and-harmony: A theory of Rogerian nursing practice. *Nursing Science Quarterly, 8,* 71-78.

Caroselli, C., & Barrett, E. A. M. (1996). *A review of the power as knowing participation in change literature.* Unpublished manuscript.

Csikszentmihalyi, M. (1996). *Creativity: Flow and the psychology of discovery and invention.* New York: HarperCollins.

Dykeman, M. C., & Loukissa, D. (1993). The science of unitary human beings: An integrative review. *Nursing Science Quarterly, 6,* 179-188.

Ference, H. M. (1986). Foundations of a nursing science and its evolution: A perspective. In V. M. Malinski (Ed.), *Explorations on Martha Rogers' science of unitary human beings* (pp. 35-44). Norwalk, CT: Appleton-Century-Crofts.

Ford-Gilboe, M., Campbell, J., & Berman, H. (1995). Stories and numbers: Coexistence without x. *Advances in Nursing Science, 18,* 14-26.

Goswami, A. (1993). *The self-aware universe: How consciousness creates the material world.* New York: Putnam's Sons.

Guba, E. G., & Lincoln, Y. S. (1989). *Fourth generation evaluation.* Newbury Park, CA: Sage.

Lincoln, Y. S., & Guba, E. (1984). The relationship between the environmental energy wave frequency pattern manifest in red light and blue light and human field motion in adult individuals (Doctoral dissertation, New York University, 1984). *Dissertation Abstracts International, 45*(7), 2094-B.

Lincoln, Y. S., & Guba, E. (1985). *Naturalistic inquiry.* Newbury Park, CA: Sage.

Morgan, G. (1983). *Beyond method: Strategies for social research.* Beverly Hills, CA: Sage.

Pedhazur, E. J. (1982). *Multiple regression in behavioral research: Exploration and prediction* (2nd ed.). New York: Holt, Rinehart and Winston.

Rogers, M. E. (1970). *An introduction to the theoretical basis of nursing.* Philadelphia: F. A. Davis.

Rogers, M. E. (1988). The science of unitary human beings: Current perspective. *Nursing Science Quarterly, 1,* x.

Rogers, M. E. (1992). Nursing science and the space age. *Nursing Science Quarterly, 5,* 27-33.

Rogers, M. E. (1994a). Nursing science evolves. In M. Madrid & E. A. M. Barrett (Eds.), *Rogers' scientific art of nursing practice* (pp. 3-9). New York: NLN Press.

Rogers, M. E. (1994b). The science of unitary human beings: Current perspectives. *Nursing Science Quarterly, 7,* 33-35.

Sondheim, S. (1984). *Sunday in the park with George: A musical.* New York: RCA Records.

5

Photo-Disclosure: A Research Methodology for Investigating Unitary Human Beings

Kaye Bultemeier

*T*he capacity of the present healthcare system to understand and respond appropriately to the diverse phenomena that people experience is limited. In response to their unfortunate situation, Rogers' Science of Unitary Human Beings provides a wholistic, nonlinear perspective for viewing human variability. The Rogerian model and appraisal tools based upon it stress the importance of descriptive research to interpret phenomena. Appraising field pattern, for example, as a natural phenomenon requires an innovative approach in the selection of methodology. Photo-disclosure, which can provide for phenomenological investigation of health concerns within a Rogerian framework, also captures personal and environmental aspects of health concerns, in order to obtain a wholistic understanding of the experience. The methodology, which combines visual and narrative data, offers an in-depth, wholistic, and personal portrayal of phenomena.

Within the current healthcare industry, the vast majority of information regarding health problems is obtained in the hospital. Certainly, the constraints associated with this site limit the type of information obtained and dictates the type of health care concerns which receive investigation. Appraisal of some health concerns, which are intermittent and do not warrant immediate attention by health care providers, has been confined to the retrospective recall of symptoms. This reliance on retrospective accounts provides limited understanding of the totality of the patient's experience.

Photo-disclosure methodology is open, providing wholistic assessment which encompasses the person and the environment. Human experiences demand examination from the perspective of the person experiencing the phenomenon. Understanding the client's perception of what is occurring to him or her is imperative if we are to gain clearer understanding of human phenomena. Photo-disclosure offers an opportunity to gain visual and narrative data which can provide such an appraisal. Multiple uses of the methodology emerge as an attempt is made to examine the lived experience of the unitary human being.

Rogers (1970) affirms "The whole of man (human beings) senses, feels, perceives, and reasons" (p. 101). Researchers can tap this sentient awareness of the person as they experience phenomena. It is through the "knowing" of the person that we gain new understanding. Self-knowing, by the client, is imperative to investigate pattern evolution from a nondisease perspective.

New research methodologies, which arise out of a homeodynamic worldview, have become essential adjuncts to investigating unitary human beings and their experiences. Rogers (1986) maintains that research in nursing must examine unitary human beings as integral with their environment, and that new research tools are needed to accomplish this task. Methodologies based upon description and explanation provide an avenue for exploration of human patterns and rhythms (Rogers, 1992). The intent of nursing research, therefore, is to examine and understand a phenomenon, and from this understanding design patterning activities that promote healing. If we are to gain a clearer understanding of lived experiences, the person's perception and sentient awareness of what is occurring is imperative. One can conclude that the life process of human beings is a phenomenon of wholeness, continuity, dynamic, and creative change. The variety of events that are associated with human phenomena provide the experiential data for research, which is directed toward capturing the dynamic, ever-changing life experiences of human beings. We are challenged to discover new and creative ways to capture health related phenomena. Selecting the correct methodology for examining persons and their environment as they are experiencing health-related phenomena is the challenge of the researcher.

METHODOLOGY DEVELOPMENT

Photo-disclosure emerges from the philosophical base of phenomenology and visual research. Both fields provide avenues for understanding the human condition. The combination of the basic elements of these research methodologies provides a new and exciting avenue to examine the human experience.

Phenomenology

Phenomenology is a methodology developed to capture an experience as it is lived (Oiler, 1986). The research occurs in the natural setting utilizing data collection methods that yield information through self-report and interviewing. The perception of the lived experience is the avenue through which the researcher gains access to the phenomenon. It is this perception that provides the data for analysis of relations and connections within related phenomena. The essential principles that guide phenomenology include attention to subjects' realities, and approaching research from a wholistic perspective while preserving the natural lived experience. The description of the lived experience is through perception, thus the experience is examined as it is lived by the subject. The researcher chooses to perceive from the vantage point of the other. Phenomenology provides a means to enter the experience of the person, and from this vantage point the experience is intuited and described.

Photographic Research

Photographic research methodologies were first used within anthropology to document cultures and events. Photographs allow the researcher to capture the phenomenon under investigation. Highley and Ferentz (1988) support the use of photographic methodologies to generate new insights and understandings of the phenomena nurses are investigating. They contend that photographs allow a nonintrusive entrance into the phenomenon and allow for repeated opportunity for evaluation of the phenomenon.

Native photography involves photographs, taken by the subject, which are used as data for interpretation. Native photography can be considered a method of nonverbal communication that provides an image for interpretation. This methodology has its origins in work done by Worth and Adair (1972) who examined movies made by Navajo Indians. Ziller (1990) changed the methodology by substituting a still-life camera for the movie camera. Ziller (1990) contends that native photography provides the ability to grasp the world through the perspective of the other, stating that through photos the researcher is able to enter the world of the subject to "see as they see" and "feel as they feel" (p. 21). Ziller developed visual phenomenology as a method for use in the examination of a variety of lived experiences. Within this process, the purpose of observation is not simply description and analysis, but understanding. Visual phenomenology allows the researcher to enter the personal experience of the subject without the researcher being physically present. When data emerge through the insider's view, via photography, the researcher becomes integral with the phenomenon and personal knowledge is achieved.

Photo-elicitation is a research methodology which has subjects respond via verbal interview to photographs of themselves, their environment, or other pictorial representation. This allows for the addition of narrative data to photographic data. The photo-elicitation process has been used extensively by anthropologists such as Collier and Collier (1990) and by sociologists such as Harper (1987). These researchers record visual images, which their subjects then verbally respond to. Within each of these processes the photo serves as a stimulus or probe to the subject.

Photo-elicitation is generally considered a verbal dialogue between informant and researcher. This methodology has been further developed by Blinn and colleagues (Blinn & Harrist, 1991; Blinn & Schwartz, 1988) who combined native photography, subject-written answers to questions about their photos, and elicitation interviews to examine phenomena. Their studies support the use of the combination of native photography with written responses by subjects concerning the photos in order to provide depth and a close native examination of the phenomenon of interest.

Photo-Disclosure

Photo-disclosure builds philosophically upon the work of Ziller within visual phenomenology and methodologically upon the written response to subject-produced photos developed and utilized by Blinn and colleagues. The intent is to use native photography along with written narrative to capture the phenomenon from the native perspective *while* it is occurring. The phenomenon is recorded pictorially and via written word simultaneously. Both methods record the same phenomenon; however, the photograph does not serve as a probe but rather provides one of two sources of data for entering and capturing the lived experience. The photographs and the words provide an active, immediate portrayal for analysis. By combining the words and the visual data, the researcher can enter into the phenomenon.

Photo-disclosure provides a native, unobtrusive entrance into the phenomenon under study. The photographs and words allow an intimate view of the phenomenon from the perspective of the subject. This native methodology captures the phenomenon when it is occurring and provides new understanding. The photo-disclosure methodology provides rich descriptive data to obtain a new understanding of phenomena.

RESEARCH UTILIZING PHOTO-DISCLOSURE

Photo-disclosure was utilized to investigate premenstrual syndrome, a common and poorly understood health concern, from a nonlinear, noncasual Rogerian perspective. The implicit variability of the female menstrual cycle has contributed to the difficulty in studying menstrually associated phenomena. The term premenstrual syndrome is used to describe variability in the female's mental and physical state associated with menstrual cycle. The existing assessment tools failed to capture the totality of the experience of women who are reporting premenstrual symptoms. Change, Rogers contends, is continuous, relative, and innovative. When change occurs, diversity is evident in the field patterning that emerges. The changing rhythmicities and patterns that evolve possess individual uniqueness. Photo-disclosure provides the opportunity to clearly describe and examine the variability of a person's experience and the change associated with the variability.

The Rogerian framework of unitary human beings provides the theoretical basis for examination of premenstrual syndrome. Perceived dissonance is the phenomenon of concern theoretically conceptualized within the Rogerian framework. Premenstrual syndrome is viewed as an exemplar of human variability manifesting as perceived dissonance (Bultemeier, 1993).

Research Question: *What are the manifestations observed and described in the photo-disclosure process when experiencing premenstrual syndrome?*

Methodology Refinement

A pilot study was conducted in two phases to test and refine the photo-disclosure methodology. The pilot studies were necessary to determine whether the methodology of photo-disclosure was appropriate for examining a health-related concern. A precedent did not exist for obtaining a unitary health-related understanding of a condition from the perspective of the client, without the presence of the health care provider.

Research Process

Twenty-one women, ranging in age from 30 to 45 years, completed the research process. The following definitions were used in this research project:

- Premenstrual syndrome day—A day selected by the subject that contained a self-defined clustering of feelings/sensations that the woman labeled as premenstrual syndrome.
- Photo-disclosure—A combination of photographs and written narrative used to capture and record a phenomenon.

Using a Polaroid instant camera, subjects took five photographs that depicted a premenstrual syndrome day and completed one photo-disclosure sheet immediately after each photograph was taken. The subjects selected the content, timing of photographs, and wrote the narrative that portrayed the phenomenon of the day.

Data Collection Procedures

The researcher met privately with the subjects in their homes, to explain the study, obtain consent, and issue materials which included a Polaroid instant camera, a 10-exposure package of film, and five photo-disclosure sheets (Appendix 5.A). Subjects were instructed not to place their name or any identifying information on the photographs or the photo-disclosure sheets and to record the data as follows: identify a day when experiencing premenstrual syndrome and on that day take five photographs which show the phenomenon, and complete one photo-disclosure sheet immediately after each photograph is taken.

A second consent form was reviewed and signed by subjects who were willing to have their photographs used for educational and research presentations. This consent was obtained after subjects had completed all phases of the data collection process so that they could have full control over their material.

Photographs and words of one subject are included to demonstrate the depth of the data collected by utilizing photo-disclosure to examine a phenomenon. These exemplars represent only a small portion of the data that were collected by this subject who will be called "Martha" (Figures 5.1 and 5.2).

Data Analysis

The analysis was conducted, by the researcher, utilizing phenomenological investigation wherein the researcher enters into the experience of the subject. A complete immersion into the phenomenon was followed by intuiting the experience and thematically coding and analyzing the data.

Figure 5.1   Martha Experiencing PMS. Martha writes: "Teeth. During premenstrual syndrome my mouth becomes a weapon. Words wound. At times, even as I am speaking I see lips moving frantically and teeth chewing at people. I know what I'm doing is hurting, but I do it anyway. Guilty."

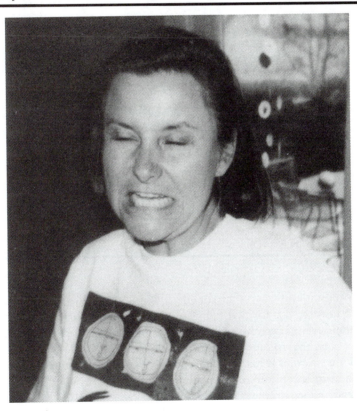

Figure 5.2   Martha Experiencing PMS. Martha writes:
"Grid locked, Me: Blocked in, boxed in (grid locked), behind,
away from. I feel so boxed in, from daily schedules and calendars
(stuck on the refrigerator and drawn in little boxes), to the house
becoming a bigger box, to the days being boxes in time.
I can't get out of the boxes."

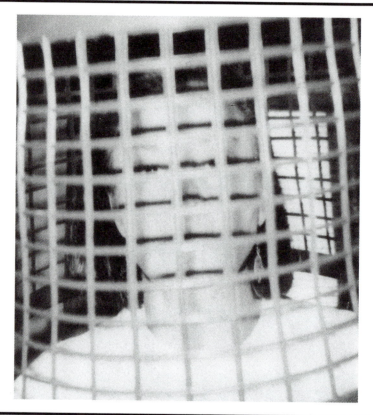

The photographs were attached to the appropriate photo-disclosure sheet. The data set formed consisted of all the photo-disclosure sheets with photographs attached depicting the phenomenon premenstrual syndrome. Data analysis involved a thematic analysis of the data set. The research question, "What are the pattern manifestations observed and described in the photographs and words of women when experiencing premenstrual syndrome?" guided the thematic analysis.

The researcher addressed the essential elements of phenomenological research: (a) bracketing of biases, (b) analyzing, (c) intuiting, and (d) describing (Swanson-Kauffman & Schonwald, 1988). Bracketing was done through the articulation of the feeling attributes of perceived dissonance. This theoretical stance was articulated and placed aside until the conclusion of the thematic analysis. Intuiting was inherent in the thematic analysis portion of the research project.

The data set was thematically analyzed following the analysis process outlined by Dobbie (1991). Data for this analysis included photos and narrative associated with Stems 1 and 2:

1. I took this photo to show . . . .
2. When I took this photo I felt . . . .

All data in the phenomenon set were considered raw data and provided access to the phenomenon. The thematic analysis proceeded in the following manner. The data were studied three times to acquire a sense of the whole. The data set of each subject, narrative with photographs attached, for all subjects, were studied in order to enter the phenomenon. Each set was intuited and reflected upon in order to gain a grasp of each individual's experience. Adjectives, nouns, and descriptive phrases were assigned to the photograph and the narrative set of each woman. The adjectives, nouns, and descriptive phrases were grouped into meaning units, and a noun was assigned to name the meaning unit. Exemplars were grouped for each meaning unit. Some exemplars represented more than one of the meaning units. When a conflict arose in grouping of the exemplar, the exemplar was grouped based upon the predominant feeling that emerged from the written narrative. A second, more refined, level of differentiating of each meaning unit was employed. The meaning units were intuited and reflected upon to uncover themes which transcended all meaning units. As the themes emerged, photographs and words combined where grouped as exemplars of the themes within each meaning unit. The data, thematically grouped within meaning units, were presented to and reviewed with three other researchers. Statements were written and a diagram was drawn that synthesized and depicted the thematic analysis. After the thematic analysis was completed, the emergent themes were reviewed and reconceptualized within the Rogerian model.

The overriding theme of the phenomenon premenstrual syndrome manifested as a feeling of disconnection. Both the words and the photographs

Figure 5.3   Diagram of PMS

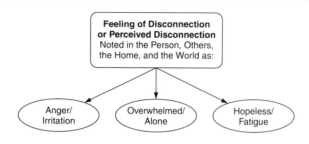

of the women revealed the sense of being disconnected. The women emerged as feeling disconnected from (a) self, (b) others, (c) their home, and (d) the world. This theme of disconnection emerged via meaning units of: (a) anger/irritation, (b) overwhelmed/alone, and (c) hopeless/ fatigue. (See Figure 5.3.)

After completion of the thematic coding, the results were explored within the Rogerian paradigm. The exploration of the results led to reconceptualization of the thematic findings as human and environmental field manifestations. Within the Rogerian perspective, the integrality of the human and environmental field provided the emergent manifestations. The manifestations were those of disconnection and disharmony. The human and the environmental field, via integrality, manifests as dissonant or nonharmonious with self, others, home, and world.

This chapter has outlined the theoretical basis for the research methodology, photo-disclosure. Additionally, the methodological process, the refinement of the methodology, the data collection procedures, and the method of data analysis are presented. The phenomenological exploration of premenstrual syndrome demonstrated the utility of photo-disclosure to examine phenomena. The methodology facilitated an open examination of the experience. This inside view provides a deeper, more intimate account of the experience. Consistent with the Rogerian nonlinear, homeodynamic model, the methodology allows clients to describe phenomena without preset limitations upon the manifestations, feelings, or the timing of the experience. Many phenomena could be more deeply understood through the utilization of photo-disclosure as a method to enter the experience of the other.

APPENDIX 5.A

Photo Disclosure Sheet

Subject number _____

Attach   Date photo taken _____

Photo   Time _____

Here   Date sheet completed _____

Time _____

Photo taken by _____

The title I would give this photo is . . . _____

_____

_____

I took this photo to show . . . _____

_____

_____

_____

When I took this photo I felt . . . _____

_____

_____

_____

Right now I wish I could . . . _____

_____

_____

_____

REFERENCES

Blinn, L., & Harrist, A. (1991). Combining native instant photography and photo-elicitation. *Visual Anthropology. 4*, 175–192.

Blinn, L., & Schwartz, M. (1988). Future time perspective: A multimethod study of how home economics students picture their lives in the future. *Journal of Vocational Home Economics Education, 6*(1), 1–17.

Bultemeier, K. (1993). *Photographic inquiry of the phenomenon Premenstrual Syndrome within the Rogerian derived theory of perceived dissonance.* Unpublished doctoral dissertation, University of Tennessee.

Collier, J., & Collier, M. (1990). *Visual anthropology: Photography as a research method.* Albuquerque: University of New Mexico Press.

Dobbie, D. B. (1991). Women's mid-life experience: An evolving consciousness of self and children. *Journal of Advanced Nursing, 16*(7), 825–831.

Harper, D. (1987). *Working knowledge.* Chicago: University of Chicago Press.

Highley, B., & Ferentz, T. (1988). Esthetic inquiry. In B. Sarter (Ed.), *Paths to knowledge: Innovative research methods for nursing* (p. 139). New York: NLN Press.

Oiler, C. (1986). Phenomenology: The method. In P. Munhall & C. Oiler (Eds.), *Nursing research: A qualitative perspective* (pp. 69–84). Norwalk, CT: Appleton-Century-Crofts.

Rogers, M. E. (1970). *An introduction to the theoretical basis of nursing.* Philadelphia: F. A. Davis.

Rogers, M. E. (1986). Science of unitary human beings. In V. M. Malinski (Ed.), *Explorations of Martha Rogers' science of unitary human beings* (pp. 3–14). Norwalk, CT: Appleton-Century-Crofts.

Rogers, M. E. (1992). Nursing science and the space age. *Nursing Science Quarterly, 5*(1), 27–34.

Swanson-Kauffman, K., & Schonwald, E. (1988). Phenomenology. In B. Sarter (Ed.), *Paths to knowledge: Innovative research methods for nursing* (pp. 97–105). New York: NLN Press.

Worth, S., & Adair, J. (1972). *Through Navajo eyes: An exploration in film communication and anthropology.* Bloomington: Indiana University Press.

Ziller, R. C. (1990). *Photographing the self: Methods for observing personal orientation.* Newbury Park: Sage.

6

Testing the Theory of Healthiness: Conceptual and Methodological Issues

Susan Kun Leddy and Jacqueline Fawcett

*I*n the Science of Unitary Human Beings (SUHB), human energy field and environmental energy field patterns change continuously and creatively through human-environment mutual process. Although the pattern that gives identity to an energy field is an abstraction, "manifestations of field patterning are observable events in the real world . . . postulated to emerge out of the human-environmental field mutual process" (Rogers, 1986, p. 6). One such manifestation is health.

Rogers does not define health, but states that "unitary human health signifies an irreducible human field manifestation" (Rogers, 1990,

This study was partially supported by a post-doctoral fellowship in psychosocial oncology awarded to Susan Leddy, Grant # T32-NR07036, Ruth McCorkle, Program Director.

p. 10) that reflects individual and societal values. The term health is derived from the root *kailo,* which signifies whole (American Heritage Dictionary, 1992). Theorists who have built on Rogers' work have defined health as "a process of becoming" (Parse, 1992, p. 35), the "experience of wholeness" (Newman, 1991, p. 224), and as "wholeness and harmony" (Carboni, 1995, p. 73).

The first author's initial conceptual work to explicate health was strongly influenced by Antonovsky's (1987) focus on the origins of health (salutogenic orientation). Antonovsky's concept of generalized resistance resources was reconceptualized as health resources, or strengths. A search of the literature revealed multiple constructs for health-related strengths, including Antonovsky's (1987) three components of coherence (meaningfulness, manageability, and comprehensibility); Kobasa's (1979) three components of hardiness (commitment, control, and challenge); and Csikszentmihalyi's (1990) conception of flow, whereby relationships with people and meaningful goals are ways in which people can have "a sense of participation in determining the content of life" (p. 4) and "a feeling of union with the environment" (p. 63). A retroductive process of reading and reflection (Hanson, 1958), led to the concept of healthiness as a health resource or strength, and an explanatory theory of healthiness.

This chapter reports the results of a test of the explanatory theory of healthiness and discusses the conceptual and methodological issues associated with the theory. The explanatory theory of healthiness (Figure 6.1) proposes that greater perceived ease and expansiveness of human-environment mutual process (participation) is associated with less perceived change. Greater participation and less change are associated with greater perceived energy, which in turn, contributes to higher healthiness. Greater participation, less change, greater energy, and greater healthiness

Figure 6.1   Explanatory Theory of Healthiness

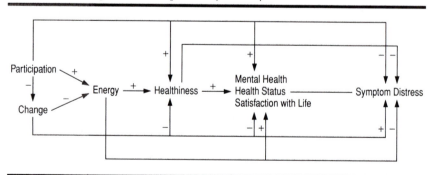

Figure 6.2   Empirically Derived Components of Healthiness

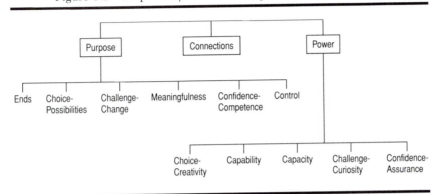

are all associated with greater mental health, current health status, and satisfaction with life, and less symptom distress.

Healthiness is defined as a state characterized by perceived purpose, connections, and the power to achieve goals (Leddy, 1996b) (Figure 6.2). *Purpose,* the perception of being energized by meaningful and significant goals, has six empirically derived dimensions: *meaningfulness,* the characterization of an aspect of the present or the desired future as having meaning, import, or value; *ends,* goals that a person aims to reach or accomplish; *challenge-change,* perceiving excitement about involvement in change toward meaningful goals; *confidence-competence,* having a belief in one's ability to accomplish goals; *choice-possibilities,* perceiving options for action; and *control,* the perceived ability to influence change.

Connections is the perception of having rewarding mutual process with others. *Power* is the perceived ability to direct energy toward the achievement of goals. Power has five empirically derived dimensions: *challenge-curiosity,* feeling comfortable with directing energy in novel ways; *confidence-assurance,* perceiving available energy as self-assurance; *capacity,* perceiving a quantity of available energy; *choice-creativity,* feeling free to direct energy; and *capability,* perceiving the ability to use or direct energy, play, and carry out activities of daily living. Healthiness is a resource that reflects a human being's perceived involvement in shaping change experienced in living.

Participation is defined as the experience of ease and expansiveness of human-environment mutual process (Leddy, 1995). Participation is a manifestation of underlying mutual process.

Change is defined as the experience of the continuous variability associated with human-environment mutual process. Change may be experienced on a continuum from facilitative (positive) to stressful and enervating (negative).

Energy is defined as the experience of dynamic and vigorous potential, in contrast with Rogers' (1990) use of the label energy to "signify the dynamic nature of the field" (p. 7).

Mental health, current health status, satisfaction with life, and symptom distress are widely accepted indicators of health. Mental health is characterized by the nature of cognitive functioning, a balance between positive and negative affect, and the extent of psychological distress. Health status is a personal judgment based on mobility and physical functioning ability. Satisfaction with life reflects a personal global cognitive value judgment about one's life. Symptom distress is the worry and anxiety associated with health problems.

METHOD

Sample

The explanatory theory of healthiness was tested using a sample of 123 ambulatory, adult volunteers, who were recruited from staff, faculty, and students of several colleges in the mid-Atlantic region; staff and board members of a community hospital; attendees at a parent-teacher meeting in the mid-Atlantic region; and by snowball convenience sampling.

The participants ranged in age from 24 to 89 ($M = 50$; $sd = 14.7$). Seventy-eight percent were female, and 99 percent were Caucasian. Forty-one percent had a college education or higher. Eighty percent were employed and 60 percent had an income above $50,000. No health problem(s)/symptom(s) were reported by 50 percent of the participants.

Instruments

The linkages between the concepts of the explanatory theory of healthiness and the instruments are shown in Figure 6.3. Healthiness was measured by the Leddy Healthiness Scale (LHS), a new, 26-item, 6-point Likert type scale (Leddy, 1996b). Participation was measured by the Person-Environment Participation Scale (PEPS), a new, 15-item, 7-point semantic differential type scale (Leddy, 1995). Change was measured by the Perceived Stress Scale (PSS), an established, 14-item, 5-point semantic differential type scale (Cohen, Kamarck, & Mermelstein, 1983). Perceived energy was measured by the Energy/Fatigue Scale (EFS), an established, 5-item, 6-point Likert type scale (Stewart & Ware, 1992). Mental health was measured by the Mental Health Index (MHI), an established, 17-item,

Figure 6.3   Linkages between Theoretical Concepts
and Empirical Indicators

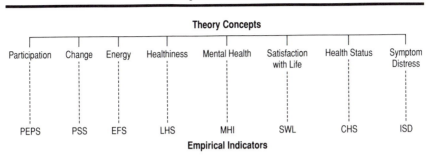

PEPS = Person-Environment Participation Scale (Leddy, 1995)
PSS = Perceived Stress Scale (Cohen, Kamarck, & Mermelstein, 1983)
EFS = Energy/Fatigue Scale (Stewart & Ware, 1992)
LHS = Leddy Healthiness Scale (Leddy, 1996b)
MHI = Mental Health Index (Stewart & Ware, 1992)
SWL = Satisfaction with Life Scale (Diener, Emmons, Larsen, & Griffin, 1985)
CHS = Current Health Scale (Stewart & Ware, 1992)
ISD = Inventory of Symptom Distress (Leddy, 1996)

6-point Likert type scale (Stewart & Ware, 1992). Current health status was measured by the Current Health Scale (CHS), an established, 7-item, 5-point Likert type scale (Stewart & Ware, 1992). Satisfaction with life was measured by the Satisfaction with Life Scale (SWL), an established, 5-item, 7-point Likert type scale (Diener, Emmons, Larsen, & Griffin, 1985). Symptom distress was measured by the Inventory of Symptom Distress (ISD), a 16-item, 5-point Likert type scale (Leddy, 1996a). In addition, one item on a background information form asked subjects to identify any health problem(s)/symptom(s). This item was scored as presence or absence of problem(s)/symptom(s). All of the instruments had adequate psychometric properties.

Data Collection Procedures

Potential subjects were approached individually, in groups, or through interdepartmental mail. The instruments, with a cover letter, a background information form, and a consent form, were mailed to volunteer subjects with a postage prepaid envelope. All instruments contained identification codes, and subjects' confidentiality was guaranteed. The study protocol was approved by a university institutional review board.

Table 6.1   Measures of Central Tendency and Variability
for the Theory Concepts

	M	SD	Potential Range	Actual Range
Participation (PEPS)	79.2	(13.8)	15–105	35–105
Change (PSS)	20.2	(7.3)	0–56	4–38
Energy (EFS)	19.9	(5.1)	5–30	5–30
Healthiness (LHS)	130.6	(15.8)	27–162	75–156
Mental Health (MHI)	82.5	(11.3)	17–102	43–102
Health Status (CHS)	28.7	(5.8)	7–35	8–35
Life Satisfaction (SWL)	26.2	(6.4)	5–35	8–35
Symptom Distress (ISD)	7.8	(6.3)	0–64	0–33

Note: See Figure 6.3.

RESULTS

Descriptive statistics for the instruments measuring the concepts of the explanatory theory of healthiness are summarized in Table 6.1.

Prior to testing the theory (Figure 6.1), the data were assessed for multicollinearity. A correlation matrix was used to examine the bivariate relationships. A magnitude greater than .80 is considered indicative of high multicollinearity (Berry & Feldman, 1985). In this study, the magnitude of the correlations ranged from .59 to .72.

The theory was then tested using path analysis. Paths were retained if the standardized beta coefficient was significantly different from zero at $p < .05$ and explained at least 5 percent of the variance in the dependent variable.

First, change was regressed on participation. Participation explained 52 percent of the variance in change, $F (1,118) = 128.71, p < .001$. Second, energy was regressed on participation and change. Participation and change explained 43 percent of the variance in energy, $F (2,117) = 45.14, p < .001$. Third, healthiness was regressed on participation, change, and energy. Participation, change, and energy explained 58 percent of the variance in healthiness, $F (3,115) = 56.21, p < .001$. The paths and standardized beta coefficients are shown in Figure 6.4.

Next, a series of path analyses were performed using participation, change, energy, and healthiness as independent variables, with mental health, current health status, satisfaction with life, and symptom distress as dependent variables. Participation, change, and healthiness explained 71 percent of the variance in mental health, $F (4,112) = 71.93, p < .001$ (Figure 6.5). Energy and healthiness explained 35 percent of the variance

Figure 6.4   Path Analysis of the Healthiness Theory
(with Healthiness as a Dependent Variable)

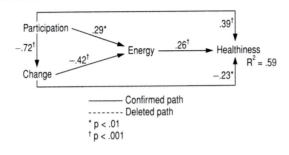

Figure 6.5   Path Analysis with Mental Health as the Dependent Variable

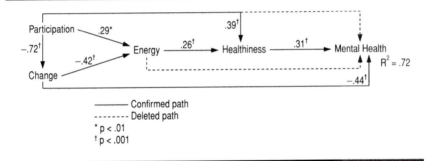

Figure 6.6   Path Analysis with Satisfaction with Life
as the Dependent Variable

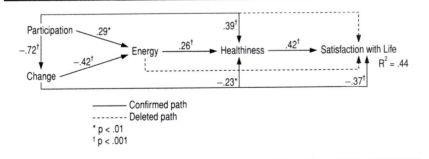

Figure 6.7   Path Analysis with Current Health Status
as the Dependent Variable

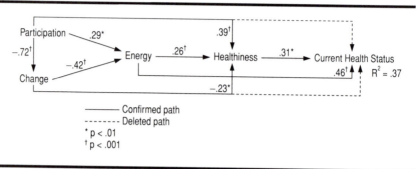

Figure 6.8   Path Analysis with Symptom Distress as the Dependent Variable

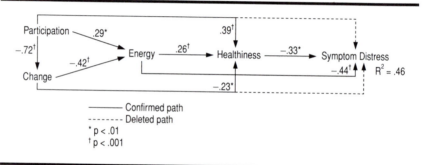

in current health status, $F_{(4,112)} = 16.57$, $p < .001$ (Figure 6.6). Change, energy and healthiness explained 42 percent of the variance in satisfaction with life, $F_{(3,115)} = 29.51$, $p < .001$ (Figure 6.7). Energy and healthiness explained 44 percent of the variance in symptom distress, $F_{(4,113)} = 23.97$, $p < .001$ (Figure 6.8).

DISCUSSION

The results of the path analysis lend initial support to the theorized relationships between participation, change, energy, and healthiness. All of the path coefficients were statistically significant, in the expected direction, and of moderate to large magnitude.

The theory that was tested proposed all possible paths from partici-pation, change, energy, and healthiness to mental health, satisfaction with life, current health status, and symptom distress. The path from participation to those variables was, however, deleted. Furthermore, the test yielded a more parsimonious theory that distinguishes the paths to current health status and symptom distress from those of mental health and life satisfaction. More specifically, the paths from change to current health status and symptom distress were deleted, and the paths from en-ergy to mental health and satisfaction with life were deleted.

CONCEPTUAL AND METHODOLOGICAL ISSUES

Rigorous conceptual and methodological work provides clarity that leads to further work. Given the rigor of the first author's ongoing work, the second author was able to identify several issues that require conceptual and methodological consideration.

The magnitude of the correlations (.59 to .72) between the scores for participation, change, energy, and healthiness suggests that these con-cepts have a common conceptual core. Within the SUHB, that common core is human-environment mutual process. Additional evidence to sup-port that interpretation comes from the correlations between power as knowing participation in change and healthiness ($r = .62$), and participa-tion ($r = .69$) (Leddy, 1996b). The magnitude of the correlations indi-cates that the concepts are not exactly the same, supporting the supposition that although mutual process is indivisible (Rogers, 1986), distinctions in manifestations are perceived by the human being.

The inclusion of participation in the explanatory theory of healthiness leads to a question about the logical congruence between the Rogerian view of mutual process and the conceptualization of participation. More specifically, given that within the SUHB, mutual process is the openness of the human and environmental field patterns and is, therefore, a constant rather than a variable, how can the conceptualization of participation as a quantifiable experience of human-environment mutual process be logically congruent with the SUHB? [Note that Rogers (1992, p. 30) maintained that there is no variance in the openness of the human and environmental en-ergy fields, explaining that "energy fields are open, not a little bit or some-times, but continuously."] The same question could also be raised about the pattern manifestations of change, energy, and healthiness. However, can the SUHB advance if relevant phenomena are not quantifiable?

The conceptual need for the concept of energy in the explanatory the-ory of healthiness also is questioned. What *is* energy? Why is the concept needed when, within the SUHB, the human and environmental fields are *energy* fields?

Moreover, the conceptual need for the concepts of mental health, current health status, satisfaction with life, and symptom distress must be questioned. How do these concepts fit into the SUHB? Are they redundant with healthiness? Have the worldviews of reciprocal interaction and simultaneous action (Fawcett, 1995) been inadvertently mixed by including these concepts in the explanatory theory?

The statistical technique used to test the explanatory theory of healthiness also must be questioned. Although path analysis is a correlational procedure, it was designed to test linear, recursive, and causal theories (Pedhazur, 1982). Despite Cowling's (1986) affirmation of correlational techniques, how can a statistical technique that tests linear, causal thinking be used within the SUHB? However, inasmuch as Rogers herself supported the test of relationships, how else can relationships be tested? Are we limited to the examination of symmetrical, that is, reciprocal, relationships by means of Pearson product moment coefficients of correlation? Or, should we eschew all inferential statistics, which reflect the reaction worldview (Fawcett, 1995), and concentrate instead on the development of qualitative methodologies that facilitate the examination of relationships?

The appropriateness of some of the empirical indicators used in this test of the explanatory theory of healthiness is clearly debatable. The Person-Environment Participation Scale and the Leddy Healthiness Scale were developed within the SUHB. In addition, although the Energy/ Fatigue Scale was not developed within the SUHB, it is consistent with the definition of energy in the healthiness theory. Moreover, the Satisfaction with Life Scale could be construed as a measure of a unitary pattern manifestation. However, the use of the Perceived Stress Scale as a proxy for negatively perceived change is conceptually weak. The Power as Knowing Participation in Change Test, which measures a unitary concept that has some overlap with change as defined in this theory, might be a better choice. The Mental Health Index, Current Health Status Scale, and Inventory of Symptom Distress, clearly measure particulate concepts of health that are not consistent with the SUHB.

The relationship of healthiness with unitary pattern manifestations should be explored. In addition, given the results of this test, it would be desirable to identify whether interventions directed at participation, change, and/or energy are associated with enhanced healthiness.

The issues raised by the test of the healthiness theory can be resolved easily—regard the SUHB not as a science but as a philosophy. If that answer were accepted, no one would have to be concerned with the problems associated with the use of quantitative methodologies. Instead, efforts could be redirected to applying the methods of philosophic inquiry to the philosophy of unitary human beings (PUHB) and the philosophy of healthiness.

If, however, that resolution is not acceptable, a substantial commitment must be made to find ways to resolve the conceptual and methodological issues raised by the articulation and testing of the explanatory theory of healthiness, which is a prototype for any explanatory theory derived from the SUHB. The two authors invite you to join them in the quest to resolve the issues.

REFERENCES

American heritage dictionary of the English language (3rd ed.). (1992). Boston: Houghton Mifflin.

Antonovsky, A. (1987). *Unraveling the mystery of health.* San Francisco: Jossey-Bass.

Berry, W. D., & Feldman, S. (1985). *Multiple regression in practice.* Beverly Hills, CA: Sage.

Carboni, J. T. (1995). Enfolding health-as-wholeness-and-harmony: A theory of Rogerian nursing practice. *Nursing Science Quarterly, 8,* 71-78.

Cohen, S., Kamaarck, T., & Mermelstein, R. (1983). A global measure of perceived stress. *Journal of Health and Social Behavior, 24,* 385-396.

Cowling, W. R., III. (1986). The science of unitary human beings: Theoretical issues, methodological challenges, and research realities. In V. M. Malinski (Ed.), *Explorations on Martha Rogers' science of unitary human beings* (pp. 65-77). Norwalk, CT: Appleton-Century-Crofts.

Csikszentmihalyi, M. (1990). *Flow: The psychology of optimal experience.* New York: Harper & Row.

Diener, E., Emmons, R. A., Larsen, R. J., & Griffin, S. (1985). The Satisfaction with Life Scale. *Journal of Personality Assessment, 49,* 71-75.

Fawcett, J. (1995). *Analysis and evaluation of conceptual models of nursing* (3rd ed.). Philadelphia: F.A. Davis.

Hanson, N. R. (1958). *Patterns of discovery.* New York: Cambridge University Press.

Kobasa, S. C. (1979). Stressful life events, personality and health: An inquiry into hardiness. *Journal of Personality and Social Psychology, 37,* 1-11.

Leddy, S. K. (1995). Measuring mutual process: Development and psychometric testing of the Person-Environment Participation Scale. *Visions: The Journal of Rogerian Nursing Science, 3,* 20-31.

Leddy, S. K. (1996a). *Development and psychometric testing of the Inventory of Symptom Distress.* Manuscript in preparation.

Leddy, S. K. (1996b). Development and psychometric testing of the Leddy Healthiness Scale. *Research in Nursing & Health, 19*, 431–440.

Newman, M. A. (1991). Health conceptualizations. In J. J. Fitzpatrick & J. S. Stevenson (Eds.), *Annual review of nursing research* (Vol. 9, pp. 221–243). New York: Springer.

Parse, R. R. (1992). Human becoming: Parse's theory of nursing. *Nursing Science Quarterly, 5*, 35–42.

Pedhazur, E. J. (1982). *Multiple regression in behavioral research* (2nd ed.). New York: Holt, Rinehart and Winston.

Rogers, M. E. (1986). Science of unitary human beings. In V. M. Malinski (Ed.), *Explorations on Martha Rogers' science of unitary human beings*. Norwalk, CT: Appleton-Century-Crofts.

Rogers, M. E. (1990). Nursing: Science of unitary, irreducible, human beings: Update 1990. In E. A. M. Barrett (Ed.), *Visions of Rogers' science-based nursing*. New York: NLN Press.

Rogers, M. E. (1992). Nursing science and the space age. *Nursing Science Quarterly, 5*, 27–34.

Stewart, A. L., & Ware, J. E., Jr. (1992). *Measuring functioning and well-being: The Medical Outcomes Study approach*. Durham, NC: Duke University Press.

7

Measurement in Rogerian Science: A Review of Selected Instruments

Juanita Watson, Elizabeth Ann Manhart Barrett, Marie Hastings-Tolsma, Linda Johnston, and Sarah Gueldner

*W*hen conducting research using Rogers' (1970, 1992) conceptual model of nursing, investigators are faced with the two questions: (1) What do I want to measure? and (2) How should I measure it? These questions were addressed by a panel of speakers at the Fifth Rogerian Conference in June 1994. Each of the authors—members of the panel—has developed an instrument to measure variables in relation to Rogers' model. A description of each one's work on her instrument is presented here.

THEORETICAL CONSIDERATIONS

Rogers' model is often perceived as being rather ethereal, "too theoretical," and somewhat difficult to capture when it comes to quantitative research and measurement. Rogers' model is highly abstract. Human beings are perceived as energy fields (see Appendix) and are said by Rogers (1992) to be infinite, pandimensional, and integral with environmental fields. The human energy field cannot be described with respect to discrete boundaries, nor in relation to spatial or temporal attributes, such as chronological age. Instead, the human energy field is identified by its unique pattern. This pattern, however, cannot be observed directly. Rather, it is revealed through manifestations of patterning that emerge from a mutual human field and environmental field process and that are "observable events in the real world" (Rogers, 1992, p. 30).

RESEARCH APPLICATIONS

Research in Rogers' model often involves identifying manifestations of patterning and developing ways of measuring them. Prior to her death in 1994, Rogers had identified some of these manifestations (see Appendix). Researchers using Rogers' model have used these manifestations as their variables, or they have used her model to develop additional manifestations of human field patterning which can be measured in research.

Barrett (1983), for example, using Rogers' idea that people participate knowingly in change, developed a theory of power and an instrument to measure this concept, the Power as Knowing Participation in Change Tool (PKPCT). Hastings-Tolsma (1992) focused on the concept of diversity and developed the Diversity of Human Field Patterning Scale (DHFSP). Johnston (1994) began with the concept of self-esteem as a self-perception concept, and after framing her ideas in relation to Rogers' model, developed the Human Field Image Metaphor Scale (HFIMS). Gueldner (1986, 1996) did some initial work with Ference (1979) on the latter's Human Field Motion Tool, the first Rogerian measurement to be developed. Her initial efforts were directed toward developing a pictorial version of Ference's instrument, but this evolved into her current work on developing the Index of Field Energy, a measure of well-being consistent with Rogerian Science. This instrument is also a pictorial tool. Watson (1993) used the manifestations of patterning identified by Rogers (1992) to study sleep-wake patterns in older women. While planning the study, it became apparent that an instrument to measure dreaming as a beyond waking experience was needed, and she subsequently developed the Assessment of Dream Experience (ADE). The remainder of this chapter is focused on the details of how these instruments were developed.

BARRETT'S POWER AS KNOWING
PARTICIPATION IN CHANGE TOOL (PKPCT)

In order to develop her instrument, Barrett (1983, 1986, 1989, 1990a, 1990b) had to first construct a power theory derived from Rogers' model. She proposed that power, like the human and environmental fields that it characterizes, can neither be directly observed nor measured. The pattern manifestations, however, that characterize power *can* be operationalized. Barrett identified these manifestations of power as (1) awareness, (2) choices, (3) freedom to act intentionally, and (4) involvement in creating changes. Using the semantic differential technique (Osgood, Suci, & Tannenbaum, 1957), she constructed a series of scales on which each of the above four concepts is rated. In an effort to avoid socially desirable responses, the word, "power" does not appear on the tool, the study participants do not know that power is the concept being investigated. For research purposes, either the total score or the four "power dimension" scores can be used.

Evolution of the PKPCT

Instrument development can be a long process, and the version of the tool initially developed is often modified based on results of subsequent studies in which the instrument is used. During the more than 13 years since the PKPCT was developed, a number of changes have been made, and the current version of the instrument is called the Barrett PKPCT, Version II (PKPCT, VII).

When the PKPCT was initially developed, content validity was established through two judges' studies, in which the judges were experts in Rogerian science and measurement. A pilot study with a national volunteer sample of 267 men and women was also conducted. Based on the results of the pilot study, the instrument was revised considerably. The modified instrument (Version I) included 48 items plus 4 test-retest items. This tool was then tested using a national volunteer sample of 625 men and women, ages 21 to 60, with a minimum of a high school education and who represented diverse occupational groups. When the scores on the PKPCT were compared with those from Ference's (1979) Human Field Motion Tool, which was also used in the study, the canonical correlation of human field motion and power accounted for 40 percent of the variance.

In the version of the PKPCT used in the pilot and initial studies, the four dimensions of power were modified by indicators of the human field (self) or the environmental field (family, occupation). No statistically significant differences were found in the pilot version or Version I of how participants responded in relation to self, family, or occupation. Thus, when Version II of the PKPCT was developed, the four dimensions of power (awareness, choices, freedom to act intentionally, and involvement in creating changes) were not modified by self, family, or occupation. Other than this, Version II was identical to Version I.

Validity and Reliability

In addition to using judges to establish content validity of the PKPCT, factor analysis has been used to evaluate construct validity. Factor loadings serve as validity coefficients. According to Nunnally (1978), factor loadings of $\geq$ .40 indicate construct validity. Factor loadings for the PKPCT ranged from .56 to .70 in the 1983 study. Trangenstein (1988), who was the first researcher to use the PKPCT in her study of 326 staff nurses, also assessed validity using factor analysis. She found a different factor structure, thus indicating a need for additional large sample studies that would continue to explore construct validity through factor analysis.

In Barrett's 1983 study, reliability of each of the four dimensions of power ranged from .63 to .99. The variance of factor scores was the method chosen to compute internal consistency. Researchers in other power studies have computed internal consistency reliability using Cronbach's alpha, and ranges have been within those found in Barrett's 1983 study. Readers are referred to the additional chapter on power in this book for specific citations where alpha coefficients for each of the power dimensions ranged from .81 to .93, and those for total power scores ranged from .94 to .97. Trangenstein (1988) reported reliabilities ranging from .86 to .92 for the power dimensions and .96 for the total power scores. The higher reliabilities for the total power scores are expected because more items are included in the reliability computation (that is 48 for the total score as opposed to 12 for each dimension score).

The four power dimensions are highly correlated with each other. This provides the empirical evidence that allows researchers to use the total power scores. One must be mindful, however, when using instruments developed in relation to particular conceptual models, the basic premises of the model cannot be violated. Since, in Rogers' model, the whole is postulated to be different from the sum of the parts, Barrett cautions users of the PKPCT that the whole of power also is different from the four dimensions of power. How once chooses which scores to use depends on what is being studied.

Uses and Issues

The PKPCT, VII has been translated into Japanese, Korean, Swedish, and Finnish. Some of the variables that have been studied along with power using both experimental and nonexperimental designs include reminiscence, creativity, feminism, spirituality, human field motion, life satisfaction, purpose in life, job diversity, job satisfaction, job involvement, anxiety, empathy, trust, and well-being. Populations studied include well adults; older adults; persons with asthma, schizophrenia, renal failure, or chronic pain; persons trying to stop smoking; post-polio survivors; women with depression; staff nurses; and nurse executives. A replication and extension of the original power study (Barrett, 1983) has been completed (Barrett, 1996).

One problem with the instrument is that scores tend to be biased upward. Questions have been raised about using quantitative methods and linear measures as tools when conducting investigations of power and other phenomena relevant to Rogers' model. While recognizing the reasons for such questions, Barrett notes that there is a value in using quantitative instruments because they may allow us to get at the answers to some theoretical questions that otherwise could not be answered at all. More details about methodological issues of the PKPCT are explored in the chapter on power in this book. Nevertheless, after over a decade of research, the PKPCT has established itself as a useful and reliable instrument in Rogerian research.

HASTINGS-TOLSMA'S DIVERSITY OF HUMAN FIELD PATTERN SCALE (DHFPS)

Hastings-Tolsma (1992) developed the Diversity of Human Field Pattern Scale (DHFPS) in order to identify the empirical indicants describing the process underlying the varying degrees of change occurring in the evolution of human potential throughout the life process. In Rogers' (1986, 1990) model, evolution of the human energy field is characterized by the creation of a more diverse pattern which manifests the nature of change. Diversity is inherent in the nature of the evolution of human field pattern. It is enhanced by the individual's capacity to participate knowingly in change. Participation in change varies and underscores the potential to design a field pattern consistent with personal preference.

Development of the DHFPS

Three theoretical dimensions had originally been proposed to constitute the variable of diversity of human field pattern. Items were developed in three categories thought to describe the construct: *statements, metaphors,* and *bipolar adjectives.* Items in all three areas were rated on a Likert-type scale. Development of the tool then proceeded in three phases. First, two judges' studies were done two months apart to establish face validity. Observer agreement of judges participating in both studies ranged from .23 to .56 for the statements, and from .44 to .55 for the bipolar adjectives. Metaphors were paired following the first judges' study, so it was not possible to determine observer agreement for the metaphors. Interrater reliability was 80 percent or better, and correlations across judges from study to study were .36 and .49 for statements and bipolar adjectives, respectively.

A pilot study was then conducted to determine whether any of the three sections of the tool measured a unitary trait. The sample consisted of 320 volunteers, ages 18 to 60. The majority (49%) were married, Caucasian (72%), and female (77%). Construct validity was assessed through principal components factor analysis for each of the three sets of items. This analysis revealed that the statements portion best captured the phenomenon under study, correlating well with the other measures in the study and also having the highest reliability coefficient (.83). Only one meaningful factor was extracted.

In an effort to establish external validity of the measure, Ference's (1979) Human Field Motion Tool (HFMT) was also administered during the pilot study. A review of the literature and the theory developed for the study suggested that the HFMT and the DHFP measure should be positively related. The statements scale was correlated moderately and significantly ($p = .001$) with the scales of the HFMT. These findings were consistent with the theory and indicated that two separate, but related constructs were measured. These findings provide support for the validity of the DHFPS, although tentative, as questions were raised about the validity and reliability of the HFMT.

Based on these studies, the 16 items comprising the statements were used as the measure of diversity of human field pattern. The items included in the statements dimension were consistent with the theoretical explanation and embodied a sense of sensitivity, self-awareness and consideration of potentials, and feature an appreciation of innovation, variety, and challenge. Thus, the unitary factor which emerged on factoring constituted the variable.

The 16 items on the DHFPS are rated in relation to a 5-point Likert-type scale. The five possible responses range from (1) strongly agree to (5) strongly disagree. Total scores are obtained by summing the ratings, and the theoretical range of scores is from 16 to 80. A *lower* total score indicates greater diversity of human field pattern.

The main study was done to determine whether the factor structure for the revised DHFPS remained stable from the pilot study. The sample for this study consisted of 173 volunteers with characteristics closely approximating those in the pilot study. Factor analysis again confirmed a unitary factor, although validity coefficients were slightly lower than in the pilot study. The reliability coefficient also was slightly lower (.81), but was at a acceptable level for a new instrument under development.

Analysis of demographic factors in relation to scores on the DHFPS revealed significant differences in scores between male and female participants ($t = 2.26$, $df = 171$, $p < .05$). Women expressed greater diversity of human field pattern than men. Significant differences also were found for those who had experienced a recent crisis ($t = 2.26$, $df = 171$, $p < .05$) and for those who meditated ($t = 2.30$, $df = 170$, $p < .05$) with both demonstrating higher means DHFPS scores.

Uses and Issues

Overall, analysis provided evidence of construct validity for diversity of field pattern, consistent with Rogers' model; however, additional methodological development is needed. Further, the development of other forms of the DHFPS may be useful and may include the use of metaphors. Certainly, the use of the DHFPS should be correlated with other Rogerian constructs, and the relative value of the instrument with different populations should be determined. The impact of culture on responses to DHFPS scores is also an important area to ascertain.

The DHFPS may have implications for clinical practice. The tool may provide a vehicle for understanding how individuals engage in the creation of desired changes. As psychometric evidence supporting reliability and validity increases, the tool should prove useful in the testing of nursing theoretical propositions, and in the examination of the extent to which selected nursing modalities foster individual health.

JOHNSTON'S HUMAN FIELD IMAGE
METAPHOR SCALE (HFIMS)

Johnston (1994), the developer of the Human Field Image Metaphor Scale (HFIMS), has indicated that she initially wanted a tool to measure self-esteem, as a self-perception concept, for use with elderly research participants. After learning about Rogers' model, however, she realized that self-esteem was too particulate a concept in relation to the holistic tenets of Rogerian science. So, in consultation with Dr. Rogers, she worked on exploring and defining the concept of Human Field Image, a term coined by Phillips (1990). Through this work, she identified two major domains of human field image: (1) perceived potential, and (2) integrality. She also developed a conceptual definition for human field image: individual awareness of the infinite wholeness of the human field.

Development of the HFIMS

The HFIMS consists of 25 metaphors which tap field potential and field integrality. Six metaphors express a strong perception of potentiality, and 12 express a positive perception of integrality. In contrast, five metaphors express a restricted perception of potential, and two express a sense of isolation. Each metaphor begins with the phrase, "I feel" and is rated on a five-point Likert-type scale. Examples of metaphors on the instrument are, "I feel one with the universe" (positive integrality), and "I feel like a worn out shoe" (negative potential). The possible range of scores on the instrument is 25 to 125. Details as to the generation and validation of the metaphors included in the HFIMS are provided in a separate article by Johnston (1994).

Uses and Issues

After the HFIMS was developed, field diversity was proposed as a correlate of human field image. A more diverse human field manifests a clearer, sharper field image, whereas a less diverse human field manifests a more blurred, indistinct image. Clarity of human field image allows the individual to more accurately perceive both the infinite and integral nature of human field image. In contrast, individuals with a blurred image may see themselves as limited in potential or enclosed by self-perceived boundaries.

The HFIMS has been shown to be a valid and reliable measure of the concept of human field image. Use of the instrument ultimately can provide valuable insights into individuals' health perceptions and health behaviors, as these are proposed to be related to perceptions of integrality and potentials. Further, it is postulated that a clear human field image is related to knowing participation in the choices and changes of life, including those related to health and well-being, whereas a blurred human field image is correlated with a passive acceptance of life experiences.

Johnston (1994) noted that further testing of the HFIMS is on-going and that this testing will expand existing knowledge related to the concept of human field image as well as that related to the Science of Unitary Human beings.

GUELDNER'S INDEX OF FIELD ENERGY (IFE)

Gueldner developed the Index of Field Energy (IFE) as a general measure of human field dynamics consistent with the Rogerian worldview. Although her initial intent was to develop a pictorial version of Ference's (1979) Human Field Motion Tool, this work evolved into the development of a separate instrument after the IFE was found to correlate almost equally not only with the HFMT (.6679), but also with Johnston's (1994) HFIMS (.6674) and Barrett's (1983) PKPCT (.7841).

Development of the IFE

The Index of Field Energy consists of 18 pairs of simple black and white line drawings, judged to represent the high and low frequency descriptors of a concept. Each pair of drawings is connected by a seven-point scale similar to that used with the semantic differential technique. Research participants are asked to indicate the point along the line that "best describes how you feel now."

Work began by taking photographs of scenes that could be interpreted in relation to Rogers' model. These were eventually converted to line drawings. Color is not used since Rogers believed color would flavor the participants' responses. The most difficult aspect of developing this instrument was the selection of pictures and drawings, as such images have different meanings to different people.

Psychometric properties of the IFE were established in two samples of 278 and 357 participants, respectively, with a final reliability coefficient of .9464 and item-to-total correlations ranging between .5023 and .8038. Factor analysis revealed two separate factors.

Uses and Issues

This pictorial instrument can be used for older adults or for adults who cannot read at a high school level. It provides a "general and user-friendly glimpse into selected manifestations of human field pattern" (Gueldner, 1996, p. 6). In addition to the paper-and-pencil version of the instrument, a game-board version of the instrument is being developed. This could be used for research participants who may have difficulty completing the written form. Work on this instrument is on-going, but it has great potential as an instrument that could be used for diverse groups of research participants.

WATSON'S ASSESSMENT OF DREAM EXPERIENCE (ADE)

Watson (1993), the developer of the Assessment of Dream Experience (ADE), indicated that the impetus for constructing her instrument arose from a desire to study sleep-wake pattern changes in older adults. Rogers' model was chosen as the framework for her study since other theories had not explained these changes, and Rogers had identified the longer sleeping/longer waking/beyond waking manifestation of patterning. To fully address this manifestation of patterning, Watson needed to determine what a "beyond waking" experience was. Rogers (1992) had indicated that meditation and paranormal phenomena were such experiences. Through a review of literature on the human sleep-wake experience, Watson posited that dreaming was also a beyond waking experience. The longer sleeping/longer waking/beyond waking manifestation of patterning was subsequently operationalized as diversity of sleep-wake rhythm and dream experience. Diversity of sleep-wake rhythm was measured using a modified Sleep Chart, but no instrument existed that could measure the experience of dreaming in a manner consistent with Rogers' model. One needed to be developed.

Development of the ADE

The Assessment of Dream Experience (ADE) is a 20-item instrument. Words used to describe dreams are rated according to a four-point, Likert-type scale. Validity of the instrument was determined through ratings of judges who were expert judges in Rogers' model and through factor analysis in an instrument development study with 100 participants. Through this latter analysis, two factors were identified and were named high diversity dream experience and low diversity dream experience. Eleven items on the instrument were designated as high diversity dream experience descriptors, whereas nine were identified as low diversity dream experience descriptors. Reliabilities for the factors were .823 and .740, respectively. The variance accounted for by the two factors was 36.8 percent. Alpha reliability of the instrument was .84.

Watson's (1993) study explored the relationships of sleep-wake rhythm, dream experience, human field motion, and time experience to further evaluate the validity of the constructs. The sample consisted of 66 healthy older women, ages 60 to 83. When scores on the ADE were assessed, the same two factors emerged on factor analysis as those in the instrument development study. Factor reliabilities and variance accounted for were also similar. It is noted, however, that the sample size should have been at least 100, especially for the factor analysis.

Uses and Issues

No difficulties were encountered in administering the instrument. Watson, however, noted that the women in her sample rated themselves as healthier, more active, and better educated than national norms. One recommendation, therefore, is that the instrument be used with larger, more diverse samples.

Watson (1993) found a statistically significant correlation between sleep-wake rhythm and dream experience scores ($r = .2945$, $p = .05$). She interpreted this as supporting the proposition that dreaming is a beyond waking experience and that diversity of sleep-wake rhythm and dream experience are indicators of change in the sleeping/waking/ beyond waking manifestation of patterning.

SUMMARY AND CONCLUSIONS

The work of several researchers in developing instruments to measure constructs in Rogers' model has been presented in this chapter. As one reviews their efforts, some commonalities can be identified and may serve as informal guides for those considering developing tools for research. First, each researcher was well-versed in Rogers' model. Anyone who undertakes instrument development in relation to any conceptual model must become thoroughly familiar with the model. This involves more than reading about the model. It is imperative that the person critically think about the Rogerian concepts and propositions, so that as ideas are brought to measurable form, the basic axioms of the model are not violated. Next, all of the researchers whose work is discussed in this chapter have strong backgrounds in research methodology and statistics. Finally, these researchers demonstrated patience in developing their instruments. Effective measurement tools are not developed "overnight" and definitive instrument development requires many studies and lots of time! These considerations should not prevent one from undertaking instrument development. As nurses become more attuned to using conceptual models to guide research, such instrument development will be essential to building nursing science.

REFERENCES

Barrett, E. A. M. (1983). *An empirical investigation of Martha E. Rogers' principle of helicy: The relationship of human field motion and power.*

Unpublished doctoral dissertation, New York University, New York. (University Microfilms No. 84-06278)

Barrett, E. A. M. (1986). The principle of helicy: The relationship of human field motion and power. In V. M. Malinski (Ed.), *Explorations on Martha Rogers' science of unitary human beings* (pp. 173-188). Norwalk, CT: Appleton-Century-Crofts.

Barrett, E. A. M. (1989). A nursing theory of power for nursing practice: Derivation from Rogers' paradigm. In J. Riehl-Sisca (Ed.), *Conceptual models for nursing practice* (3rd ed., pp. 207-217). Norwalk, CT: Appleton-Century-Crofts.

Barrett, E. A. M. (1990a). An instrument to measure power as knowing participation in change. In O. Strickland & E. Waltz (Eds.), *The measurement of nursing outcomes: Measuring client self-care and coping skills* (Vol. 4, pp. 159-180). New York: Springer.

Barrett, E. A. M. (1996). *The relationship of human field motion and power: A replication and extension.* Manuscript in preparation.

Ference, H. M. (1979). *The relationship of time experience, creativity traits, differentiation, and human field motion.* Unpublished doctoral dissertation, New York University, New York. (University Microfilms No. 80-10281)

Gueldner, S. H. (1986). The relationship between imposed motion and human field motion in elderly residents living in nursing homes. In V. M. Malinski (Ed.), *Explorations on Martha Rogers' science of unitary human beings.* Norwalk, CT: Appleton-Century-Crofts.

Gueldner, S. H. (1996). Index of field energy. *Rogerian Nursing Science News, 8*(4), 6.

Hastings-Tolsma, M. T. (1992). *The relationship among diversity of human field pattern, risk taking, and time experience: An investigation of Rogers' principles of homeodynamics.* Unpublished doctoral dissertation, New York University, New York. (University Microfilms No. 92-337755)

Johnston, L. W. (1994). Psychometric analysis of Johnston's Human Field Image Metaphor Scale. *Visions: The Journal of Rogerian Nursing Science, 2*(1), 7-11.

Nunnally, J. C. (1978). *Psychometric theory* (2nd ed.). New York: McGraw-Hill.

Osgood, C. E., Suci, C. J., & Tannenbaum, P. H. (1957). *The measurement of meaning.* Chicago: University of Illinois Press.

Phillips, J. R. (1990). Changing human potentials and future visions of nursing. In E. A. M. Barrett (Ed.), *Visions of Rogers' science-based nursing* (pp. 13-25). New York: NLN Press.

Rogers, M. E. (1970). *An introduction to the theoretical basis of nursing.* Philadelphia: F.A. Davis.

Rogers, M. E. (1986). Science of unitary human beings. In V. M. Malinski (Ed.), *Explorations on Martha Rogers' science of unitary human beings* (pp. 4-23). Norwalk, CT: Appleton-Century-Crofts.

Rogers, M. E. (1990). Nursing: Science of unitary, irreducible, human beings: Update 1990. In E. A. M. Barrett (Ed.), *Visions of Rogers' science-based nursing* (pp. 5-11). New York: NLN Press.

Rogers, M. E. (1992). Nursing science and the space age. *Nursing Science Quarterly, 5*(1), 27-34.

Trangenstein, P. A. (1988). *Relationships of power and job diversity to job satisfaction and job involvement: An empirical investigation of Rogers' principle of integrality.* Unpublished doctoral dissertation, New York University, New York.

Watson, J. (1993). *The relationships of sleep-wake rhythm, dream experience, human field motion, and time experience in older women.* Unpublished doctoral dissertation, New York University, New York. (University Microfilms No. 94-11208)

Part Three

Traditions of Mysticism and Rogerian Science

8

Mysticism in Buddhist Philosophy and Rogerian Science: Awareness, Integrality, and Compassion

Effie S. Hanchett

Mystical experience constitutes one thread of the rich tapestry of Rogerian science's tradition of theory, research, and practice. In the Rogerian worldview, beyond waking experiences are one manifestation of field patterning in unitary human beings (Rogers, 1990, p. 9). In Rogerian research, "the unitary human being's direct experiencing of the mutual process of field interaction . . . [was] a unifying theme of the studies" presented in Malinski's book (1986, p. 189). Meehan (1990) described the importance of a state of meditative awareness for the practice of therapeutic touch.

The direct experience of an active, everchanging, interrelated, compassionate universe is one way of considering mystical experience and has commonalities with both Rogerian science and the Middle Way

Consequence School of Tibetan Buddhist philosophy. Four aspects of mystical experience emerge from this definition: awareness, activity, interrelatedness, and compassion. All are addressed in Rogerian science and in Buddhist philosophy.

AWARENESS

Awareness is inherent in both Rogerian science and Buddhist philosophy. Rogerian science describes sleep, wake, and beyond waking experiences as manifestations of field patterning in unitary human beings (Rogers, 1992b). Many Buddhist texts define awareness (consciousness) and describe methods for developing it in detail.

Rogerian Science

In Rogerian science, "experience is meant in the broadest sense, and not just mere sensory experience. . . . The experience of pattern manifestations is accompanied by perception. Perception means that the person has the capacity to be aware to some degree of pattern manifestations" (Cowling, 1990, p. 52). Beyond waking experiences reflect what might traditionally be called states or levels of consciousness. Rogerian science based studies have explored mystical experience (Cowling, 1986) and relationships between manifestations of mystical experience, such as a sense of oneness with nature, experiences of timelessness, and peak experiences (Barrett, 1986; Ference, 1986; Miller, 1985).

Buddhist Philosophy

Consciousness and awareness, synonymous in Tibetan Buddhist philosophy, are defined as "that which is luminous and knowing" (Gyatso, 1988, p. 49). They are not the mind of a sentient being, but rather they are momentary, active agents of knowing, aspects of the mind. There are two ways of valid knowing—direct perception and inference. Direct perception is knowing without any intervening concepts. It is immediate, changing in concert with an everchanging reality. No time is spent in formulating labels or mental images (Gyatso, 1994). That which a person experiences by means of direct perception cannot be adequately expressed in words. Direct perception may or may not conform with reality. However, direct *valid* perception is, by definition, nonmistaken. There are three types of direct valid perception—sensory, mental, and direct yogic (the meditator's perception).

Direct sensory perception is the knowing that emerges from sense faculties, sense organs, and sense powers in concert with the specific thing perceived. Nurses appraise clients by sensing subtle cues, such as skin color, odors, tone of voice, or the sound of breathing. These cues are perceived and synthesized so rapidly that the expert is unaware of the specifics of the cues or the process. The nurse knows only that something about the client is different, and that it is important.

Direct mental perception includes clairvoyant knowing. Clairvoyant knowing includes seeing or hearing at a distance and knowing others' minds. It is manifested in the clear and salient urge to call a relative or client when you have no logical reason to do so—and finding out the reason after you call.

The direct perception of selflessness (the lack of a self that exists independently of others) is one step in the meditator's development of consciousness. The direct perception of the interdependent arising of all persons and phenomena is the meditator's ultimate goal in the development of consciousness. This nonconceptual knowing of the interdependent process of the universe as a whole is a capacity present in all sentient beings. Things seem, however, to exist in some solid independent way; we believe it and do not notice the interrelated momentary changes that are always occurring.

Rogerian Science and Buddhist Philosophy

Rogers' (1990, 1992a) manifestations of field patterning address awareness. Rogers identified multiple manifestations of awareness in her statement that "abstraction and imagery, language and thought, sensation and emotion are fundamental attributes of . . . humanness" (1970, p. 67). Similarly, Cowling (1990) stated the "knowledge derived from pattern information involves multiple modes of awareness by the nurse" (p. 53).

Buddhist philosophy also addresses many manifestations of awareness. Both conceptual and nonconceptual awareness are significant in the development of consciousness. Buddhist descriptions of direct mental and yogic perception are similar to Rogerian science's description of awareness as a manifestation of diverse field patterning emerging from the mutual process of infinite human and environmental energy fields.

ACTIVITY

The idea of activity pervades both Rogerian science and Buddhist philosophy. The dynamic nature of the energy field in Rogerian science and the gross and subtle change which characterize all reality in Buddhist philosophy suggest similar perspectives.

Rogerian Science

Activity permeates the key definitions and principles of Rogerian science. The energy field, dynamic in nature, is in continuous motion. Integrality, reasonancy, and helicy (see Appendix) describe an active field process. Barrett's concept of power, "the capacity to participate knowingly in the nature of change. . . . describes the way human beings interact with their environment to actualize some potentials for change rather than others" (Barrett, 1990, p. 108).

Buddhist Philosophy

Activity also permeates Buddhist philosophy. It includes both gross (observable by ordinary human sense organs) and subtle (unobservable by ordinary human sense organs) actions of body, speech, and mind. The definition of consciousness, "that which is luminous and knowing" (Gyatso, 1988, p. 49), describes knowing as an activity. Activity is also inherent in the concept of dependent arising (also translated as interdependent origination) which is the continuous emergence of phenomena in interrelationship with a multitude of everchanging "causes and conditions" (Napper, 1989).

Rogerian Science and Buddhist Philosophy

Buddhist philosophy separates human actions into those of body, speech, and mind. Rogerian science does not. Activity is continuously present in both systems, occurring at observable levels and in ways that are too rapid or too subtle as to be seen directly by the human eye.

INTERDEPENDENCE AND INTEGRALITY

The principle of integrality in Rogerian science describes a mutual process of human and environmental fields (see Appendix). The principle of dependent arising in Buddhist philosophy describes the ultimate nature of reality as a continuously emerging interrelated process. It is always in flux as the constellation of factors, that is the pattern of interrelationships, is continuously changing.

Rogerian Science

The mutual human and environmental field process describes the logical "relationship" between person and environment. The individual and his or her own unique environment are engaged in a mutual process. Meaning provides one example of that process. Bohm and Sheldrake (1986) spoke of innumerable possible dimensions of meaning. Reeder (1984) presented the idea of past as remembered and future as anticipated within the experience of the now. In the mutual process of person and environment, meaning emerges as a pattern manifestation. A person's experience and ways of being are manifested in his or her environment. At the same time, the pattern of the environment is manifested in the person's experience.

Madrid's (1990) description of caring for Roger, a terminally ill patient with AIDS provides a powerful description of that mutual process. The decorations in Roger's hospital room, the greeting cards and flowers from family and friends, were manifestations of his love and care for others, their love and care for him, and the significance of his friends and family to him. Madrid's care included Therapeutic Touch as a healing modality through which the quality of the human and environmental field unfolded to create a diverse pattern whereby he deliberately and knowingly participated in change.

The mutual process of human and environmental fields is a continual process of dynamic, subtle action. Through this process, the caregiver's experience manifests the experience of the one cared for, and the one being cared for manifests the experience of the caregiver. The client's sorrow, depression, hope, or joy is experienced by the healthcare provider. Similarly, the provider's perceptions and feelings are experienced by the client. Perceptions and feelings emerge from the mutual process of the unified field of the client-provider dyad and their environment. It is also through this process that the client knowingly participates in change whereby healing and the peaceful acceptance of impending death emerges.

Buddhist Philosophy

The principle of dependent arising (interdependent origination) of the Middle Way Consequence School of Tibetan Buddhist philosophy asserts that nothing has solid, independent existence. "A doer arises dependent on a doing. And a doing depends on a doer." Everything in the universe is interrelated. Napper (1989), described it as follows:

> *Things arise dependent on causes and conditions, they gain their identities in relation to other things. Nothing stands alone, autonomous and*

isolated, but instead exists only in a web of interconnectedness. Like near and far, all things are relative, ... Things are always in flux, always changing; there are no independent autonomous entities. (p. 3)

The web of reality *is* simultaneous action, nothing more, nothing less. That does not mean that, for example, you or your client do not exist, or that you cannot act to influence the direction of change. But it does mean that noting exists independently of its atoms, our attributions, or all the activities of others that contribute or have contributed to its existence.

The philosophy of the Middle Way Consequence School of Tibetan Buddhist philosophy is based on that of Nagarjuna, Chandrakirti, and other Middle Way Indian scholars. The central principle is the assertion that nothing exists independently. Things exist, but they exist like the reflection of the moon in water. The reflection is real. We are moved by its beauty. Any sane person with his or her vision intact would agree that the reflection is there. However, it depends on the moon, the stillness of the water, and the clarity of the sky for its existence. Similarly, the moon, the water, the sky exist only in interrelationship with a myriad of other factors. Each of those other factors also exists only in interrelationship. Nothing exists independently of the net of interrelatedness.

Rogerian Science and Buddhist Philosophy

Both Rogerian science and Buddhist philosophy describe the manifestations of patterning, reality as we perceive it, as emerging from a dynamic process. Some translators of Buddhist philosophy identify multiple "causes and conditions" in this process. Rogerian science denies causality.

COMPASSION

"The purpose of nurses is to promote health and well being for all persons wherever they are" (Rogers, 1994, p. 28). In Buddhist philosophy, compassion is defined as the wish that all living beings "be freed from suffering" (Gyatso, 1988, p. 168). It is the ultimate motivating force for action.

Buddhist Philosophy

In Buddhist philosophy, compassion is a quality of consciousness. It does not discriminate between someone who is seen as one's best friend, and someone who is seen as one's enemy. Moreover, as awareness increases, indifference decreases. Even beings unknown to self are part of the web of existence and included within the field of compassion and awareness (Gyatso, 1988).

Compassion sees the suffering aspect of all sentient beings, motivates one to develop consciousness to see reality as it is, and enables one to heal others (Tayang, n.d./1984). It arises from seeing and experiencing the suffering of oneself and others and creates an overriding determination to eliminate it. Great compassion involves taking upon oneself the burden of freeing all sentient beings from suffering and joining them with happiness.

Rogerian Science

Martha Rogers stated (1994), "the science of unitary human beings provides the knowledge for potential for imaginative and creative promotion of the well-being of all people" (p. 35). Compassion, in the sense of the desire that all people be free from suffering and free to achieve their maximum potential, has been such a basic assumption of Rogerian science that there was little explicit discussion about it. Discussions were about how (not whether or why) to achieve well being for all. I remember a spirited discussion with Martha in the 1970s in which she exhorted us, in our committment to social justice, not to be indifferent to the suffering of middle class suburbanites. "They suffer, too," she said.

The overriding drive to relieve suffering is a hallmark of true compassion. Rogers (1992b) stated, "The pressing need to study people in ways that would enhance their humanness has coordinated with the accelerating technological advances and forced a search for new models" (p. 28). According to Rogers, "the purpose of nurses is to promote health and well-being for all persons wherever they are" (p. 28).

There is no clearer manifestation of compassion than the great respect for the individuality of each person that is the logical consequence of the principle of helicy, and the search for the goodness and forces for growth, no matter how expressed, in each person, that are at the heart of Rogerian science. The search is not to identify clients' "problems" but rather to become aware of their unique pattern manifestations as experiences of desired goals and challenges to be met in attaining them.

Buddhist Philosophy and Rogerian Science

Indian and Tibetan Buddhist traditions describe meditative techniques to build understanding of our debt of gratitude to all beings through recognition of the extent of our interrelatedness. Rogerian science emphasizes the value of the unique paths and expressions of the drive for increasing awareness and diversity of each individual, family, or community. The well-being of others is the purpose for action in both systems. Compassion is dealt with explicitly and extensively in Buddhist philosophy. It is the ground from which Rogerian science emerged and although more implicit than explicit, pervades its principles, research, and practice.

CONCLUSION

Rogerian science and Buddhist philosophy address all of human experience. Mysticism as the compassionate awareness of the active, ever-changing, interrelated and compassionate universe is central to Buddhist philosophy. Rogerian science includes studies of mysticism and Rogerian practice includes the art of practice modalities grounded in meditative states of awareness. Buddhist philosophy describes ways to develop compassion and direct, nonconceptual awareness of a continuously emerging, interrelated universe. Rogerian science identifies the human and environmental field process, awareness as one of its manifestations, and values the uniqueness of the individual and his or her own manifestations of increasing diversity. Rogerian science is manifested in scientific study of mystical phenomena. Rogerian practice modalities incorporate this knowledge for the purpose of human betterment.

REFERENCES

Barrett, E. A. M. (1986). Investigation of the principles of helicy: The relationship of human field motion and power. In V. M. Malinski (Ed.), *Explorations on Martha Rogers' science of unitary human beings* (pp. 173-184). Norwalk, CT: Appleton-Century-Crofts.

Barrett, E. A. M. (1990). Health patterning with clients in a private practice environment. In E. A. M. Barrett (Ed.), *Visions of Rogers' science-based nursing* (pp. 105-115). New York: NLN Press.

Bohm, D., & Sheldrake, R. (1986). Matter as a meaning field. In R. Weber (Ed.), *Dialogues with scientists and sages: The search for unity* (pp. 105-123). New York: Routledge & Kegan Paul.

Cowling, W. R. (1986). The relationship of mystical experience, differentiation, and creativity in college students. In V. M. Malinski (Ed.), *Exploration on Martha Rogers' science of unitary human beings* (pp. 131-141). Norwalk, CT: Appleton-Century-Crofts.

Cowling, W. R. (1990). A template for unitary pattern-based nursing practice. In E. A. M. Barrett (Ed.), *Visions of Rogers' science-based nursing* (pp. 45-65). New York: NLN Press.

Ference, H. M. (1986). The relationship of time experience, creativity traits, differentiation and human field motion. In V. M. Malinski (Ed.), *Explorations on Martha Rogers' science of unitary human beings* (pp. 95–106). Norwalk, CT: Appleton-Century-Crofts.

Gyatso, L. (1994). *The four noble truths* (S. Gyatso, Trans.). Ithaca, NY: Snow Lion.

Gyatso, T. (1988). (J. Hopkins, Trans.). *The Dalai Lama at Harvard.* Ithaca, NY: Snow Lion.

Madrid, M. (1990). The participating process of human field patterning in an acute-care environment. In E. A. M. Barrett (Ed.), *Visions of Rogers' science-based nursing* (pp. 93–104). New York: NLN Press.

Malinski, V. M. (1986). Afterword. In V. M. Malinski (Ed.), *Explorations on Martha Rogers' science of unitary human beings* (pp. 189–191). Norwalk, CT: Appleton-Century-Crofts.

Meehan, T. C. (1990). The science of unitary human beings and theory-based practice: Therapeutic touch. In V. M. Malinski (Ed.), *Explorations on Martha Rogers' science of unitary human beings* (pp. 67–81). Norwalk, CT: Appleton-Century-Crofts.

Miller, F. A. (1985). The relationship of sleep, wakefulness and beyond waking experiences: A descriptive study of M. Rogers' concept of sleep-wake rhythm. *Dissertation Abstracts International, 46,* 116b.

Napper, E. (1989). *Dependent arising and emptiness.* Boston: Wisdom.

Reeder, F. (1984). Philosophical issues in the Rogerian science of unitary human beings. *Advances in Nursing Science, 6*(2), 14–23.

Rogers, M. E. (1970). *An introduction to the theoretical basis of nursing.* Philadelphia: F.A. Davis.

Rogers, M. E. (1990). Nursing: Science of unitary, irreducible, human beings: Update 1990. In E. A. M. Barrett (Ed.), *Visions of Rogers' science-based nursing* (pp. 5–11). New York: NLN Press.

Rogers, M. E. (1992a). Nursing science: A science of unitary human beings. *Rogerian Nursing Science News, 4*(3), 7.

Rogers, M. E. (1992b). Nursing science and the space age. *Nursing Science Quarterly, 5*(1), 27–34.

Rogers, M. E. (1994). The science of unitary human beings: Current perspectives. *Nursing Science Quarterly, 7*(1), 33–35.

Tayang, L. L. (1984). *One hundred and eight verses in praise of great compassion* (J. I. Cabezon, Trans.). Mysore, India: Mysore. (Original work published n.d.)

9

Hindu Mysticism: The Realization of Integrality

Barbara Sarter

*M*ysticism is rooted in an experience and perception of essential unities. Although it is a universal human experience, its expressions and rationales are formed by whatever intellectual or religious tradition a person is attached to. In this chapter I will introduce the reader to the Hindu expression of mysticism and discuss how Hindu mystical insight resonates with and affirms the Science of Unitary Human Beings, a contemporary paradigm for healing. The links between mysticism and healing will be illuminated through this comparative analysis of an ancient mystical tradition and a modern healing paradigm.

There is no single central source of Hindu dogma. There are few rituals or beliefs common to all Hindus. In fact, the distinguishing characteristic of Hinduism is its sincere acceptance of all forms of worship and spiritual belief as legitimate avenues to the ultimate goal of union with the divine.

The goal of the soul's journey in Hindu mysticism is the union of the personal self with the universal self.

THE UPANISHADS

The Upanishads present the deepest insights of the ancient sages of India, and are held in highest reverence by Hindus. The word "upanishad" means "sitting near," and denotes how these texts were revealed and recorded (Radhakrishnan & Moore, 1957). The disciples of the rishis, the wise men of ancient India, sat near their gurus in the forest to receive these teachings.

Brahman and Atman

Two concepts are fundamental to Upanishadic philosophy: brahman and atman. Brahman denotes the universal, ultimate reality, the first principle of the universe, which creates, supports, and also destroys the material universe. Atman is the inner self of each individual, the soul, that which remains when all that is not our essential nature is eliminated (Radhakrishnan, 1953). The key point of Upanishadic philosophy is that brahman and atman are, in essence, identical. Their seeming separation and difference is an illusion created by the human mind. Since they are ultimately one, we know brahman by coming to know our innermost self, atman. Tat tvam asi, "that art thou," is the fundamental truth revealed in the *Upanishads* (Deussen, 1966).

An ontology of consciousness is essential to explain the unity of brahman and atman. The ultimate reality, the substance of the universe, is consciousness. Brahman is sat-chit-ananda, existence-consciousness-bliss (Dasgupta, 1959). Power, knowledge, and joy reach their fullest manifestation in this ultimate reality. Since the universe is made of brahman, all within it, from atom to human, is also consciousness at various levels of development. Our innermost self, atman, is consciousness, the subject which perceives objective reality (Saksena, 1971).

Being and Becoming

Some Upanishadic texts maintain that as pure consciousness, the ultimate reality is also pure being; that is, it is changeless and transcends space and time (Ranade, 1968). The becoming aspect of the world, change within the framework of space and time, is maya, illusion. But others maintain that the ultimate reality is also pure becoming; that, in fact, being and becoming are aspects of one reality. Watts (1963) discusses extensively this unique characteristic of Hindu mysticism—the unity of opposites, the reconciliation of the dualities that plague Western thought. In modern Upanishadic commentaries, the duality of being and becoming (or spirit and matter) is resolved by a view that consciousness and energy are the same substance. Energy is conscious, and consciousness is energy or force (Ramananda, 1953; Aurobindo, 1970). The question inevitably arises in the mind of the mystic who has experienced the infinite peace of change-less being, "Why becoming at all? Why this world of change and all that goes with change—pain, fear, suffering, desire?" The *Upanishads* answer that it is the divine lila, the play of the infinite, to differentiate into sepa-rate and changing units. It is simply the nature of the ultimate reality (Ra-mananda, 1953). At the beginning of the universe, the changeless being evolves itself into the manifest cosmos, and its multifarious units, from quarks to humans, begin to evolve back into itself. Suffering is due to our sense of separation from others and from the infinite. It facilitates the evolution of consciousness toward its ultimate reunion with brahman (Ramananda, 1953).

THE BHAGAVADGITA

The Bhagavadgita is the most widely read spiritual text among Hindus. Though it derives its main ideas from the *Upanishads,* it abandons the abstract philosophy of its roots and emphasizes the personal and ethical aspects of the individual's relation with the infinite (Radhakrishnan & Moore, 1957). It is presented as a dialogue between Krishna, an incarna-tion of the divine, and Arjuna, his disciple, as Arjuna faces his own rela-tives as enemies in a battle between good and evil. In this scripture, Krishna explains the three paths of yoga, all of which are means to con-sciously accelerate the speed of the soul's evolution back to its source in the ultimate reality. The three yogas are devotion, work without desire, and knowledge of the ultimate truth.

In his teachings to Arjuna, Krishna refers to the body as a field, and the soul as the knower of the field. The body is the field in which all events—birth, growth, death—occur. The consciousness that observes these events as a witness is the knower of the field (Radhakrishnan & Moore, 1957). Thus, there is an apparent dualism between matter and spirit. *The Bhagavadgita* is a deeply poetic expression of the mystical insights of Hinduism, "Arjuna, I am the Self seated in the heart of all beings; so I am the beginning and middle and also the end of all beings" (*The Bha-gavadgita,* Chapter 10, Verse 20).

MEDITATION IN HINDU MYSTICISM

In Hindu spiritual discipline, there are two fundamentally different approaches to meditation, although the goal in both is the same—the merging of individual consciousness with the supreme consciousness. Ramananda (1966) calls these the paths of ascent and descent. The path of ascent requires strict control of the mind and the senses so that the personal consciousness can be raised to its highest levels. The path of descent, however, requires complete relaxation and openness of body and mind, so that the supreme consciousness can easily permeate the individual.

The closeness of the seeker with the guru or spiritual guide accelerates the transformation of consciousness. This closeness is not necessarily a physical proximity, but is based on a strong connection which transcends space and time. The guru provides the seeker with a *mantra,* a special energy-endowed sound grouping (Ramananda, 1966). The power of the mantra lies within its sound and its meaning. It dissolves the boundaries of the ego and invokes union with its source. The mantra of greatest power will be that which comes from the supreme itself. Such mantras are used today by those who are initiated into Hindu mystical paths.

THE SCIENCE OF UNITARY HUMAN BEINGS

Martha Rogers developed the Science of Unitary Human Beings over a period of three decades (Rogers, 1970, 1980, 1987, 1990, 1994). It is a conceptual framework for nursing practice based on a new world view of synthesis and holism. Open energy fields replace atoms as the building blocks of the universe. Energy fields are infinite, without boundaries, and are identified by their pattern. This is an evolutionary science in which field pattern is constantly changing, becoming more diverse (the principle of helicy). Pattern is also changing from lower to higher energy frequencies (the principle of resonancy). This paradigm for healing "studies, holistically, human beings as energy fields" (Rogers, 1994, p. 4). Person, the human energy field, and environment, the environmental energy field, are integral. They cannot be separated and are in a continuous mutual process of change (the principle of integrality). Reality itself is pandimensional; it is nonlinear and infinite (Phillips, 1994).

Ideas of causality and predictability are rejected in the Science of Unitary Human Beings. Open energy fields are spontaneous and self-organizing. Though they change into increasingly diverse patterns, the exact nature of change cannot be predetermined. This does not, however, imply that human beings can only passively undergo whatever is happening. Knowledgeable participation in change is possible, for sentience (self-awareness) is a manifestation of the human energy field.

The goal of healing in the Science of Unitary Human Beings is to promote well-being of the person by increasing the harmony of the person-environment process and by facilitating the human field's conscious participation in its movement toward increasing diversity and higher frequencies. Barrett (1986) has developed and researched the concept of power as the person's capacity for knowing participation in change. Increasingly this capacity is an important goal of this healing science. Healing may occur right up to and beyond the dying process, for the human field, being infinite in a pandimensional reality, does not cease to exist after death of the body. It has evolved into a frequency higher than the senses can perceive (Phillips, 1990).

HINDU MYSTICISM AND THE SCIENCE OF UNITARY HUMAN BEINGS

Recent discussion among Rogerian scholars has explored the implicit spirituality of the Science of Unitary Human Beings (Phillips, 1994), a topic which seems to have "come out of the closet" in the last few years. This modern healing paradigm resonates with the insights of ancient mystical traditions. I will now explore some of these areas of resonance, pointing out certain areas of dissonance, with Hindu mysticism.

The integrality of the human and environmental fields can be seen as a contemporary expression of the essential unity of atman and brahman. Rogers maintains that we are integral with the environmental field, which is pandimensional and not bounded by space or time. In the *Upanishads,* the cosmic environment is brahman, the manifest universe as well as the unmanifest deeper reality underlying it. Atman, the personal self, is differentiated, individuated brahman. There is a personal self, but it is ultimately one with brahman. In both systems, then, the individual, though differentiated, is one with a larger reality. Realization of this truth is an important step toward healing in Rogerian science, and toward liberation in the mystic.

The changing pattern of the human and environmental energy fields correlates with the becoming aspect of reality in Hindu mysticism. The supreme reality displays complete creativity and freedom in its dance of becoming (Watts, 1963). This is congruent with Rogers' rejection of causality and insistence on the unpredictability of change. However, the Hindu believes that in the manifest universe of the involved infinite, change is governed by the law of karma, in which for each action there is a reaction (Ramananda, 1953). The interplay of action and reaction stimulates the evolution of consciousness, whose final goal is the union of atman and brahman. In Rogerian terms, this evolution of consciousness is indeed a movement toward increasing diversity. It can also be called a movement toward increasing health.

In Rogerian science, there is no changeless aspect of reality. This is a clear area of disagreement with Hindu thought. The ontological assertion of a changeless reality has a long history in both Western and Eastern philosophy. Ramananda (1953) explains its logic in the following way, "Being is the necessary basis of Becoming. Becoming is impossible without the support of Being. The phenomenal world could not be without a changeless stay. Being is like the invisible point which is woven into the form of this mighty universe" (p. 22). It is conventional in Hindu thought that space and time are considered dimensions relevant to the world of becoming; change can only occur within space and time (Deussen, 1966). Being, the changeless reality, transcends space and time. Rogers' assertion of a changing reality that is not bound in space and time is philosophically unique.

Rogers (1988) postulated the theory of accelerating evolution, which maintains that the rate of change in the universe is increasing as evolution progresses. The philosophy of yoga maintains that the pace of the evolution of consciousness can be hastened. There are some very interesting connections between what Rogers calls the manifestations of relative diversity in field patterning (Rogers, 1990) and the characteristics of the advanced practitioner of yoga. For example, some manifestations of increasing diversity are a sense of timelessness and a state of awareness that moves from longer waking to beyond waking. It is well known that accomplished yogis (practitioners of yoga) sleep very little and are often in what are called higher states of cosmic consciousness when they are awake (and even when asleep). A visionary awareness which is more penetrating than imagination is also a manifestation of increasing diversity. Such an awareness has been documented in numerous accounts of the lives of saints, prophets, and mystics throughout the ages and from all traditions. Mystical awareness meets the criteria for increasing diversity, and therefore accelerating evolution, of the human field. Phillips (1994) refers to this awareness from a Rogerian perspective as *pandimensional awareness,* an awareness which transcends space and time, mind and body.

The body is called a field in *The Bhagavadgita,* and the soul the knower of the field. The entire person is called an energy field in the Science of Unitary Human Beings. Soul would be categorized as a manifestation of field pattern in Rogerian thought (Rogers, personal conversation, 1993), as would the consciousness it holds of itself and its world. But

Rogers has always avoided involvement in theological discussion, she has been careful to maintain a scientific approach to analysis of the human energy field.

Meditation has been discussed and researched extensively by Rogers and scholars of her science (Rogers, 1994). It is promoted as a non-invasive, energy-based modality for nursing practice. The Hindu theory of mantra as an energy-endowed sound is entirely congruent with the Rogerian view of meditation. According to the principle of resonancy, the mantra will be in mutual process with the human field and a higher wave frequency will occur, accelerating the evolution of the field. The phenomenon of mantra warrants careful investigation by Rogerian scientists as a potentially powerful healing therapy.

To summarize the link between Rogerian science and Hindu mysticism, I will postulate how the mystic will be described from a Rogerian perspective. The Hindu mystic experiences integrality and resonance with the highest, most subtle frequency energies, perceives a pandimensional awareness, and exhibits manifestations of accelerating evolution and increasing diversity of field pattern. The goal of healing in the Science of Unitary Human Beings is to accelerate evolution through harmonious human/environmental process. Mysticism, then, becomes an avenue to true healing.

REFERENCES

Aurobindo, S. (1970). *The life divine* (6th ed.). Pondicherry, India: Sri Aurobindo Ashram Trust.

Barrett, E. A. M. (1986). Investigation of the principles of helicy: The relationship of human field motion and power. In V. M. Malinski (Ed.), *Explorations on Martha Rogers' science of unitary human beings* (pp. 173–184). Norwalk, CT: Appleton-Century-Crofts.

The Bhagavadgita [The song divine] (22nd ed.). Gorakpur, India: Gita Press.

Dasgupta, S. (1959). *Hindu mysticism.* New York: Frederick Ungar.

Deussen, P. (1966). *The philosophy of the Upanishads.* New York: Dover.

Phillips, J. (1990). Changing human potentials and future visions of nursing: A human field image perspective. In E. A. M. Barrett (Ed.), *Visions of Rogers' science-based nursing* (pp. 13–25). New York: NLN Press.

Phillips, J. (1994). The open-ended nature of the science of unitary human beings. In M. Madrid & E. A. M. Barrett (Eds.), *Rogers' scientific art of nursing practice* (pp. 11–25). New York, NLN Press.

Radhakrishnan, S. (1953). *The principle Upanishads.* New York: Harper.

Radhakrishnan, S., & Moore, C. A. (1957). *A sourcebook in Indian philosophy.* Princeton, NJ: Princeton University Press.

Ramananda, S. (1953). *Evolutionary spiritualism.* Hardwar, India: Sadhana Karyalaya.

Ramananda, S. (1966). *Adyatmik sadhan* [A manual on spiritual endeavor] (Vol. 1). Bisalpur, India: Sadhana Karyalaya.

Ranade, R. D. (1968). *A constructive survey of Upanishadic philosophy* (2nd ed). Bombay, India: Bharatiya Vidya Bhavan.

Rogers, M. E. (1970). *An introduction to the theoretical basis of nursing.* Philadelphia: Davis.

Rogers, M. E. (1980). Nursing: a science of unitary man. In J. Riehl & C. Roy (Eds.), *Conceptual models for nursing practice* (2nd ed., pp. 329–337). New York: Appleton-Century-Crofts.

Rogers, M. E. (1987). Rogers' science of unitary human beings. In R. Parse (Ed.), *Nursing science: Major paradigms, theories, and critiques* (pp. 139–146). Philadelphia: Saunders.

Rogers, M. E. (1988). Nursing science and art: A prospective. *Nursing Science Quarterly, 1,* 99–102.

Rogers, M. E. (1990). Nursing: Science of unitary, irreducible human beings: Update 1990. In E. A. M. Barrett (Ed.), *Visions of Rogers' science-based nursing* (pp. 5–11). New York: NLN Press.

Rogers, M. E. (1994). Nursing science evolves. In M. Madrid & E. A. M. Barrett (Eds.), *Rogers' scientific art of nursing practice* (pp. 3–10). New York: NLN Press.

Saksena, S. K. (1971). *Nature of consciousness in Hindu philosophy* (2nd ed.). Delhi, India: Motilal Banarsidass.

Watts, A. (1963). *The two hands of God: The myths of polarity.* London: Rider.

10

Mysticism/Spirituality of Aborigine People and Rogerian Science

Francelyn Reeder

*A*boriginal people (also known as "The Real People") of Australia have a saying that spirits are just visiting this earth (Arrien, 1993), and this sentiment is depicted in a photograph taken by Martha Brahmley of Martha Rogers donning a baseball cap inscribed with the words "Just Visiting This Planet." Humor always carries a kernel of truth. Martha's worldview is linked with that of the aboriginals, the oldest continuous human inhabitants on the earth (40,000 years) (Crumlin & Knight, 1991).

Although Martha E. Rogers has left this planetary life to continue on perhaps into another form of eternal life, her influence can still be felt by anyone who is open to her. Space nursing was an alien concept when introduced by Martha Rogers. It is not simply a teaching tool to stretch one's imagination beyond the old worldview. Reports of encounters with aliens from outer space are increasing in frequency by persons who say they have had encounters with these aliens. Spectators attempt to make what is strange more familiar. Aliens and abductants are strange because they have never been experienced. Another group of inhabitants on the earth have been described as "alien" in stories by Marlo Morgan (1991) in her recent book, *Mutant Message*. She unfolds her firsthand experiences with "The Real People" in the Outback of Australia. Morgan's stories are so "other worldly" they still taunt me to ask, am I a mutant with a message from spirits of the heavens and inner earth? Is Martha Rogers among those spirits? If any of us are foot-dragging mutants of the Western old worldview, we may be those invited daily by our ancestors in the spirit world to wake up to new realities toward becoming *real human beings!*

I will share an analysis and weaving of stories illuminating unique and common features between Aboriginal spirituality and Rogerian science, a science long recognized as expressing a more inclusive, expansive worldview than traditional Western science. These features are best recognized through approximations of six qualities:

1. The animating origins of thought;
2. The nature of reality being lived or described;
3. The process of learning in becoming a human being;
4. The nature of human and environment relationships;
5. The belief in and participatory nature of creative potential for celebration; and
6. The purpose of the authors' system of thought and life.

"Aborigine" is used synonymously here with the term "indigenous people." Angela Arrien (1993), a Western anthropologist and folklorist, tells us "when we listen to land-based peoples, we are listening to our oldest selves" (p. 7). Change and healing, transition, and rites of passage are supported by indigenous cultures through mythic structures, and the incorporation of art, science, music, ritual, and drama into daily life (Eliade, 1964). Every culture in the world sings, dances, and tells stories, and these are practices to which we all have access (Ingerman, 1991). Arrien attempts in her research to understand Shamanic otherness. She reports that Shamanic traditions draw upon the power of four archetypes in order to live in harmony and balance with the environment and with our own inner nature. As Arrien (1994) describes it, the four-fold way pervasive of indigenous people consist of the Warrior, the Healer, the Teacher, and the Visionary.

UNIQUENESS AND COMMONALITIES

The Animating Origins of Thought

Vision is central to the spirituality of Indigenous People. In some native cultures of America, the Sacred Hoop is synonymous with the term "authenticity: being connected with one's spirituality." In the words of Black Elk, "I was seeing in a sacred manner the shapes of all things in the spirit, and the shape of all shapes as they must live together, like one being; and I saw that the sacred hoop of my people was one of many hoops that made one circle, wide as daylight and as starlight, and in the center grew one mightily flowering tree to shelter all the children of one mother and one father" (Black Elk, 1990). Rogerian science expresses unity and diversity through the principle of integrality.

The *visionary* Shamanic tradition expresses the name attributed most frequently to Dr. Rogers. The Shaman advises, "If you do not express your own original ideas, if you do not listen to your own being, you will have betrayed yourself" (Arrien, 1993, p. 84). Rogers' work is at the frontiers of knowledge where seeing is from *being there,* with a vision, and having the courage to write it down for others to see (Malinski & Barrett, 1994). Singing—giving voice to the vision—is common to Shamanic visions. I do not recall hearing Dr. Rogers singing or chanting, but she certainly went on vision quests, awakening evermore to life's purpose and her own original medicine common to Shamans. The Shaman learned to trust vision and intuition by spending times of solitude in nature remembering and claiming one's creative spirit. Dr. Rogers seemed to be able to find solitude in the middle of New York City as did Shaman Gabrielle Roth of urban life (1989). The noise of the busy city was not a distraction, but the frequency, rhythm, and energy of human beings in complexity was more like music to her ears; no doubt Martha knew the secret of participating knowingly with the diversity and complexity, as she was open to see new emergents, continuously and innovatively manifesting. Nonetheless, the family cottage in Pigeon Forge in the Smokey Mountains of Tennessee and Phoenix in the desert of Arizona were primary environments for Martha's nature vision quests. The Shamanic visionary is the truth teller. Dr. Rogers was certainly not weak hearted! She stayed within the Sacred Hoop of vision and spoke out with courage and well-placed humor.

Aboriginal artists (Crumlin & Knight, 1991) have commented that Western artists actively use their imagination to create art. In contrast, Aboriginal artists *first* receive a message from their ancestors in the spirit world and then express this sacred message through painting, dancing, singing, drumming, and other creative expressions. Rogers also began with a vision of reality that she then communicated to the discipline of nursing through a life of exquisitely imaginative, erudite writing. Rogers' refinement of her own language continued to the end while her vision notably endures. One of Rogers' goals was to awaken people to wonders of the world! Both Aboriginal people and Rogerian science are ordinary, beginning with cosmic insight, engaged in the deep structures of reality.

The Nature of Reality Being Lived or Described

The nature of reality lived by the Aborigine is powerfully told by Marlo Morgan through a story in *Mutant Message,* after she spent a four-month "walkabout" with a small tribe in Australia. The guides to life are the invisible spirits of the earth in their nomadic wanderings in the desert. Aborigine People are amazed at the Westerners' addiction to "form," expressed in seeking and believing only concrete reality. Rogerian science describes the nature of the human-environment relationship through the principle of integrality in *non-causal* terms, without spatial or temporal attributes (Malinski & Barrett, 1994). The nature of unitary human beings is also nonlinear, evolutionary, and innovative toward greater complexifying diversity. Rogers makes an existential claim in saying unitary human beings *are;* they do not *have,* energy fields! Energy fields describe the dynamic nature of the human-environmental mutual process, disclaiming the static forms of the old Western world view. Aborigines also express a belief in a dynamic, unfolding world (Arrien, 1994).

The Process of Learning in Becoming a Human Being

The processes of learning in becoming human beings for both Aboriginal people and Rogers are those that engage in intuition, imagination, telepathy, and other paranormal processes of communion of humans and environment, coextensive with the universe. A knowing participation, not limited to logical categories of space-time distinctions, gives rise to story telling. Metaphors which preserve the context and process of unfolding and becoming human are common ways for the Aboriginal people to remind generations of the mystery, beauty, grace, and dignity of who we really are. Angela Arrien tells the story of the Ubian woman, also known as "The Necklace" story. The story is retold again and again and invites the listener to notice: When did you come into the story? When did you resist the story? Listeners pay attention to the teaching meant for them today in the story. The storytellers are the "memory keepers." The memory of your people is intimately connected with remembering who you are! This involves "soul work," a deep continuous journey of becoming human.

Rogers preserved the gift and joy of story telling in a way that either moved the listener to a comfort level of awareness and connection with it, reducing anxiety about her world view; *or* told stories that would awaken people to current trends in society that needed action *by* the profession of nursing. I believe this expressed Rogers' moral sense of responsibility and accountability as a human being sharing the abundance of this planet and the universe.

The Nature of Human and Environment Relationship

The nature of the human environment relationship expresses the Aboriginal reality of all actual experiences, and possibilities and potentialities of happenings on their journey toward becoming human beings; and similarly expresses the nature of change in the mutual process of becoming unitary human beings described in Rogerian science. Further, the nature of this relationship of humans in Mother Earth and Father Sky is expressed in "dream time" walkabouts following the song-lines and footprints of their ancestors who crossed the land before them. The oneness of all people of the earth is beyond tribes, skin color, ethnicity, and beyond all categories or names the Western scientists give them (Harner, 1993). Several stories can be told from the experiences of Marlo Morgan depicting the unfolding of life in dream-time in the walkabout that is the best illustration of *telepathic communion* with nature I have ever read! She gave examples of becoming water to find water! The pandimensionality of life definitely transcends space and time and yet is vitality itself and awakened life at its best!

Rogerian science presents a worldview of pandimensionality, integrality, helicy, and resonancy undergirded with nonspatial, nontemporal attributes of a mutual process of human and environmental fields. The reference to waking and beyond waking, and the movement of awareness from imaginative to visionary, is similar to the world view of Aboriginal ways of "seeing" the life process. The latter kind of seeing is beyond sense and imagination, given for the first time and qualitively, indistinguishably emerges from all time.

The Belief in and Participatory Nature of Creative Potential for Celebration

Aboriginal people express the participatory nature of their creative potential in thanksgiving ceremonies and celebrations. It is common when the people have lost spirit or soul to be asked these questions: When did you stop dancing? When did you stop singing? Illness and disease are thought to relate to life choices; a failure to use one's gifts and talents by not expressing voice and body vitality. Soul work is expressed through costumes of favorite animal spirits that, danced in ceremonials, create the spirit they enact while benefiting the whole community. Drumming expresses the earth-human heartbeat, which keeps the vibrant rhythm of life flowing. Touching each other while looking with clear open eyes, as unspoken messages are given through telepathy, is common practice within celebrations of becoming, healing, and receiving gifts for being more fully human. Marlo Morgan, for example, was invited to a ceremony by "The Real Tribe" and to receive the gift of dream-time seeing, so that she could ask and receive what she needed to survive her walkabout. Such communing with Mother Earth and Father Sky leads inevitably to finding symbols of guidance in the animal and natural worlds. For Morgan, her sighting of a raven and the appearance of a wolf at dawn were particularly important. She received these signs and others with gratitude and trust in a timeless movement forward "toward forever!" Rogerian science postulates a mutual process of human-environment that is evolutionary, innovative, and unpredictable, a stance which invites us to be open to surprise and to unexpected manifestations of patterns. Such patterns are the signs and symbols that appear and point to the unfolding of creative potential continually expressing itself in the life process. Rogers invites *us* to celebrate life in all its forms, even through death to new life, including her own.

The Purpose of the Authors' System of Thought and Life

The purpose of these two systems of thought and life, the Aboriginal and Rogerian, illuminate their differences most clearly in the ways they actually enhance each other. The spirituality of the Aborigine as well as the Navajo Native American Indian, for example, is expressed from generation to generation as a lived reality, for the purpose of communicating their traditions in the ways of becoming real human beings. The teachings are given in concrete, experiential detail through story telling. Soul retrieval happens through recognizing oneself in the stories, and the context of these stories which evoke infinite possibilities and memories. Another way to express the uniqueness of the Aborigine system of life is that it provides the "content" of life as living unfolds.

The purpose of Rogerian science as a system of thought and life is to describe the *nature* of the *invisible* reality (nonspatial-nontemporal-nonlinear), and to illuminate the *nature* of human-environment reality recognized through pattern seeing, a way of seeing that will lead scholars to a freedom from old ways of seeing the world, and to participate knowingly from a vision that requires the fullest expression of human-environment creative potential; that is, to get on with life in its evolutionary, innovative, ultimate expression. Rather than the content of the world, the *patterns* of a reality are thus implicated by Rogerian science's principles of homeodynamics, as a body of nursing knowledge, and point the way to becoming creative human beings. Spirituality may merely be a euphemism if not envisioned as integrality of the pandimensionality of all the living and non-living, no matter where they are! With passion—compassion is born of a profound respect for all that exists and struggles into becoming! (McGaa, 1990).

REFERENCES

Arrien, A. (1993). *The four-fold way: Walking the paths of the warrior, teacher, healer and visionary.* San Francisco: Harper San Francisco.

Arrien, A. (Speaker). (1994). *Gathering medicine* (Tapes 1 & 2). Boulder, CO: Sounds Tape Recording.

Black Elk, W., & Lynn, W. S. (Eds.). (1990). *Black Elk: The sacred ways of a LaKota.* San Francisco: Harper San Francisco.

Crumlin, R., & Knight, A. (Eds.). (1991). *Aboriginal art and spirituality.* North Blackborn, Victoria: Collins Dove, HarperCollins.

Eliade, M. (1964). *Shamanism: Archaic techniques of ecstasy.* Princeton, NJ: Princeton University Press.

Harner, M. (1993). *The way of the shaman* (3rd Ed.). San Francisco: Harper San Francisco.

Ingerman, S. (1991). *Soul retrieval: Mending the fragmented self through shamanic practice.* San Francisco: Harper San Francisco.

Malinski, V., & Barrett, E. A. M. (Eds.). (1994). *Martha E. Rogers: Her life and her works.* Philadelphia: F. A. Davis.

McGaa, E. E. M. (1990). *Mother Earth spirituality: Native American paths to healing ourselves and our world.* San Francisco: Harper San Francisco.

Morgan, M. (1991). *Mutant message.* Summit, MO: Marlo Morgan.

Roth, G. (1989). *Maps to ecstasy: Teachings of an urban shaman.* Novato, CA: Nataraj.

Part Four

Patterns of Rogerian Knowing in Theory and Research

11

Pattern Appreciation: The Unitary Science/Practice of Reaching for Essence

W. Richard Cowling III

*P*attern appreciation is both a way of unitary knowing and an approach to the development of unitary nursing science and practice. Earlier work of the author on a template and guiding assumptions for unitary nursing practice (Cowling, 1990, 1993a) led to further refinement of the concept and the process. Pattern appreciation is logically derived from the concepts and principles of the Science of Unitary Human Beings (Rogers, 1992). Pattern appreciation has been used to integrate practice and research into a unitary model of science/practice. The critical features of pattern appreciation as synoptic, participatory, and transformative are used in reaching for the essence of pattern.

THE CONCEPT

A guiding template for research and practice was developed using appraisal of the human field pattern as one feature (Cowling, 1990). The term *appraisal* has a central meaning associated with evaluation and estimation. To appraise is "to fix a price for, assign a money value to" (Oxford English Dictionary, 1994). The concept of appreciation was chosen as an alternative because the meaning was broader and encompassed the features of being fully aware or sensitive to or realizing; being thankful or grateful for; and enjoying or understanding critically or emotionally (American Heritage, 1985, p. 121). The following elemental characteristics of appreciating were derived from a critical review of the Oxford English Dictionary (1994) definitions of appreciation:

1. Perception of the *full* force.
2. Sensitive to and sensible of *delicate impression or distinction*.
3. Perception, recognition, and intelligent notice.
4. Expression of one's estimate.
5. Sympathetic recognition of excellence.
6. Gratefulness, enjoyment, and understanding.

These distinguishing characteristics are embraced in the unitary conceptualization of appreciation. While it is clear that appraisal and appreciation are related, appreciation can be differentiated by these features or characteristics. It appears that the intent and focus of appraisal is evaluating and estimating. The intent and focus of appreciation is extended and expanded to perceiving, being aware of, sensitive to, and expressing the full force and delicate distinctions of *something* while sympathetically recognizing its excellence as experienced in gratefulness, enjoyment, and understanding. The *something* in unitary science and practice terms is energy field pattern.

APPRECIATION AND THE SCIENCE
OF UNITARY HUMAN BEINGS

The concept of unitary pattern appreciation is unique to the Science of Unitary Human Beings. It was developed and evolved with the intention of creating a way of doing science and practice from a unitary perspective. It is both a way of knowing from a unitary ontological perspective and an essential attitude toward persons as energy fields. Unitary pattern appreciation is capturing the essence of pattern emergent from human/environmental fields beyond any focus on a part or a summation of the parts. It is not possible to observe energy field pattern directly (Rogers, 1992), nor is it possible to capture pattern directly. Pattern appreciation is differentiated from formal operations thinking and systems thinking and is the path of unitary thinking.

Pattern appreciation is consistent with the conceptual system known as the Science of Unitary Human Beings (Rogers, 1992). "Pattern is a key postulate in this system. It is defined as the distinguishing characteristic of an energy field perceived as a single wave. Pattern is an abstraction, its nature changes continuously, and it gives identity to the field. Moreover, each human field pattern is unique and is integral with its own unique environmental field pattern" (Rogers, 1992, p. 30). These statements specify the major conceptualizations within Rogers' framework: pattern, energy field, openness, and pandimensionality.

Pattern

Pattern appreciation, as a process of science and practice, accepts the centrality of pattern as the distinguishing characteristic of an energy field. To appreciate pattern, one is required to be sensitive to and sensible of the distinction of a human energy field. This involves accepting the uniqueness of each human field pattern and its own unique integral environmental field pattern. The perception, recognition, and intelligent notice of pattern and its full force are also consistent with the framework because it emphasizes the whole rather than particulars.

Energy Fields

Appreciation is sensitivity to the human as an energy field arising from noticing, perceiving, and recognizing its delicate distinctions. Energy is neither good nor bad in and of itself, yet as a patterned field it exhibits qualities that distinguish its uniqueness. As will be described later in detail, the process of appreciation involves expressing an estimate and sympathetically recognizing excellence. The expression of estimate is one that reflects the essence of pattern and could take a variety of forms specific to the practice and/or research. The idea of estimate here is one of worth; pattern has some worth or some purpose for that individual, thus its inherent excellence.

Openness

Appreciation rests on the assumption that while one cannot directly know another's field, openness provides the context for mutuality that shared fields can be perceived through sensitivity and sensibility. Openness is also the grounds for the integral nature of human/environmental fields. Thus openness is the grounding context for mutual sharing that is essential to pattern appreciation as process. "A universe of open systems explains the infinite nature of energy fields, how the human and environmental fields are integral with one another, and that causality is invalid" (Rogers, 1992, p. 30). Openness, infinity, integrality, and the absence of causality are inextricably intertwined in the concept of pandimensionality.

Pandimensional

Pandimensional is "a nonlinear domain without spatial or temporal attributes" (Rogers, 1992, p. 29). Pandimensionality has been described by Rogers (1992, p. 31) as "a way of perceiving reality." Further, "the term pandimensional provides for an infinite domain without limit" (Rogers, 1992, p. 31). This is also the grounds for an ontological view of acausality and unpredictability as reflective of the nature of change. Moss (1995) points out that "causality ceases the moment we become referent to infinity" (p. 66). From this perspective, "the universe and human beings are revelation happening" (Moss, 1995, p. 66). From the view of infinity, "there is no definite causal explanation for our suffering or for our joy. Certainly we suffer, but we are not merely victims. We are that which is transformed in the suffering. Nothing is frozen; everything is unfolding, evolving" (Moss, 1995, p. 67).

Thus with pattern appreciation, there is the awareness of infinity from an orientation of sympathetic recognition of excellence and gratefulness, enjoyment, and understanding. Moss (1995) puts it more clearly, "The present is always infinitely potential, always as fresh and ripe with inception as the very moment of the Big Bang or the birth of life from the archaic seas billions of years ago. The present is ever ready to surprise us with a movement and a possibility we can never really imagine and never fully control. This is precisely our dread—and the good news" (p. 67). So pattern appreciation is being referent to both pattern and to infinity or pandimensionality.

Principles of Homeodynamics

The three principles of homeodynamics (Resonancy, Helicy, and Integrality) together postulate the nature and direction of human/environmental field pattern change (Rogers, 1992). Rogers notes that pattern reveals itself through manifestations that are continuously innovative. Evolution of life is "a dynamic, irreducible, nonlinear process characterized by increasing complexification of energy field patterning" (Rogers, 1992, p. 31). The nature of change is characterized by diversity and unpredictability. Continuity of change is perceived as a rapid wave frequency that appears to the observer as a single, unbroken event. Field pattern diversity is viewed as relative for an individual. Marked increase in diversity exists between individuals as well. Rogers (1992) claims that this perspective of field pattern diversity makes individualization of nursing services explicit.

Pattern appreciation is an orientation to humans that recognizes the need for individualization of nursing. By perceiving, recognizing, and taking intelligent notice as well as being sensitive to and sensible of the relative distinctions in human field pattern manifestations, the scientist and practitioner can express more clearly and deeply the nature and direction of change. Capturing the complexification of energy field patterning is essential to the development of unitary nursing science and practice.

ART AND SCIENCE: PROCESS, ORIENTATION, APPROACH

Pattern appreciation is a process, an orientation, and an approach for research and practice. Pattern appreciation has the potential to serve the purposes of an integrated practice/scientific endeavor that leads to both practice and scientific knowledge simultaneously.

Process

Pattern appreciation is a process of reaching for the essence of pattern. As Rogers (1992) has noted pattern that cannot be accessed directly but can be revealed through its manifestations. Sources of pattern information are conceptualized in this appreciation perspective as experience, perception, and expression. "Humans are constantly and contiguously all-at-once experiencing, perceiving, and expressing, providing the source for human field pattern appreciation" (Cowling, 1993a, p. 202). Humans are manifesting pattern in the form of experience, perception, and expression simultaneously as a singular continuous event.

Experience is the raw encounter of living loaded with sensation. The basic assumption is that one is capable of experiencing what one is manifesting; in this case pattern manifestations. Experience is viewed as "any item or ingredient within our stream of consciousness" (James, as cited in LeShan & Margenau, 1982). The Oxford English Dictionary (1994) offers two defining aspects of experience vital to its understanding. One is the actual observation of events considered as a source of knowledge and the second is the fact of being consciously the subject of a state or condition. Experience involves the rawness of living through sensing and being aware as a source of knowledge.

"Perceiving is the apprehending of experience or the ability to reflect while experiencing" (Cowling, 1993a, p. 202). Perception also involves making sense of what is going on in experience. The conscious knowing aspect of experience is perception in the midst of experience; the two cannot be disentangled. Perception is also defined by the concept of personal observation (Oxford English Dictionary, 1994). The critical features of perception are awareness, apprehension, personally observing, and making sense of experience. If one is able to experience one's pattern and its manifestations, then perception is conscious knowledge of pattern. Thus, perceiving is essential to knowing participation in change described by Rogers (1992).

Expression is the manifestation of experience and perception which is reflective of human field pattern (Cowling, 1993a, p. 202). The Oxford English Dictionary (1994) defines expression as "the action or process of manifesting" which is the substance of this conceptualization. "Expressions of pattern form the informational substance for pattern appreciation" (Cowling, 1993a, p. 203). Expressions are any data form that comes forward in the encounter of the scientist/practitioner and client/participant. Expressions are essentially energetic manifestations of field pattern. Expressions are not pattern itself; rather "pattern is grasped only in and through its expressions" (Cowling, 1990, p. 53).

Pattern appreciation requires an inclusive view of what counts as pattern information. Expressions include sensations reported as well as observables. Sensations might include meditative insights, rapid or slow heartbeats, movement, time passage, shifting change, sadness, dreams, and concerns. Observables could be gait, posture, activity level, muscle strength. Pattern information is energetic manifestations that are expressed in many forms. "In essence, anything expressed is relevant to unitary pattern since humans are unitary creatures" (Cowling, 1993a, p. 204).

The act of doing pattern appreciation is essentially the same within the context of a scientific endeavor and a practice endeavor. However, purposes may differ with each endeavor. Pattern appreciation offers a way of unitary knowing that extends previous ways of knowing associated with systems thinking (Cowling, 1993b). Pattern appreciation can be useful for generating practice knowledge and/or theoretical knowledge either separately or simultaneously. Pattern appreciation used for purposes of practice would be aimed at assisting an individual with pattern exploration in relation to a client-centered goal. In this context, a pattern appreciation engagement may lead to some deeper understanding that may guide actions of the client. In the scientific endeavor the purpose might be to generate scientific knowledge specific to that individual pattern and disseminate findings to a wider audience of scholars. In this case the emphasis is on conceptual and theoretical development specific to that unique pattern. This conceptual and theoretical knowledge also may have immediate practice implications as well. Both endeavors use pattern appreciation as a way of understanding pattern information (expressions or energetic manifestations) from a unitary perspective. The two endeavors may be intertwined in a scientific/practice endeavor.

Rogers (1992) has argued that "a theoretically sound foundation that gives identity to nursing as a science and an art requires an organized abstract system from which to derive unifying principles and hypothetical generalizations" (p. 28). She further explained that "a science may be defined as an organized body of abstract knowledge arrived at by scientific research and logical analysis. This knowledge provides a means of describing and explaining the phenomena of concern" (p. 28). In pattern appreciation, the phenomena of concern are experience, perception, and expressions that are energetic manifestations of pattern. Understanding is sought in the context of and specific to the unique human field pattern. "Unifying principles and hypothetical generalizations" that guide action for that particular individual may be explicated. However, given a broader interpretation of Rogers' case for "unifying principles and hypothetical generalizations," it may be possible to investigate some identified phenomenon using pattern appreciation and look for these unifying principles and hypothetical generalization across individuals with relative pattern appreciation profiles that could inform the scientist about the phenomenon. Additional support for this perspective is implied by Rogers' (1992) statements concerning the applicability of a science of unitary human beings to groups. The group energy field "may be a family, a social group, or a community" (p. 30). Perhaps in this case it may be a group of respondents in a pattern appreciation study.

The process of pattern appreciation derives from the orientation made explicit in guiding assumptions of unitary knowing for practice and research (Cowling, 1990, 1993a, 1993b) and the explicit features of pattern appreciation. The process unfolds specifically in congruence with the individual situation and the purposes of the participants involved. Pattern appreciation is also an art form for using knowledge creatively in practice.

Orientation

The orientation of unitary pattern appreciation is based on refinement of guiding assumptions (Cowling, 1993a, pp. 201–209):

1. The basic referent of nursing science and practice is human energy field pattern.
2. Human field pattern is appreciated through manifestations of the pattern in the form of experience, perception, and expressions.
3. Pattern appreciation requires an inclusive perspective of what counts as pattern information (energetic manifestations).
4. Knowledge derived from pattern appreciation involves multiple modes of awareness by the scientist/practitioner.

5. A construction process of synopsis and synthesis is requisite to unitary knowing for pattern appreciation.

6. Various formats for presenting and conveying pattern appreciation are applicative to the unitary perspective.

7. The primary source for verifying pattern appreciation and profile is the participant.

8. The basic foundation for purposive nursing strategies and for design of research is the participant's knowing participation in change.

9. The concepts and principles of unitary practice and science for the individual participant emerge from pattern appreciation and approaches are determined by the participant.

10. The concepts and theoretical knowledge derived from pattern appreciation reflect unique patterning of participant.

Unitary pattern appreciation by its conceptual refinement implies the following orientational features:

1. Pattern appreciation seeks for a perception of the full force of pattern.

2. Pattern appreciation requires sensitivity to and sensibility of the pattern manifestations that give identity to each person's unique pattern.

3. Pattern appreciation involves perception, recognition, and intelligent notice of human expressions that reflect pattern.

4. Pattern appreciation takes the form of an estimate of unitary energy field pattern in the form of pattern profile construction.

5. Pattern appreciation implies sympathetic recognition of excellence of energy field pattern meaning that pattern is significant regardless of characteristics.

6. Pattern appreciation is approached with gratefulness, enjoyment, and understanding that reaching for essence of pattern has potential of deepening understanding in service to individual and knowledge development for practice and science, and ultimately transformation of participants.

Approach

The approach of pattern appreciation serves both science and practice simultaneously in a scientist/practitioner model. These are the elements proposed in such a model of pattern appreciation:

1. The scientist/practitioner seeks engagement with another for purposes of exploring unitary human field pattern. It is also possible that another will seek the scientist/practitioner for exploration and deeper understanding of unitary human field pattern. Both are considered equal co-participants in these endeavors.

2. Specific intentions of scientist/practitioner are made explicit to the participants through a mutually derived and negotiated informed consent process.

3. The participants co-create form and structure for engagement for pattern appreciation. This can take the form of interviewing, observing, and creative expressions or any combination of these.

4. Documentation of experience, perceptions, and expressions are accomplished through such means as journaling, audio and/or visual recording, photographing artifacts offered by the participant, recordings of music that reflects pattern information, and actual creative products of the engagement such as drawings, music, poetry, and so on.

5. Journaling for the scientist/practitioner may involve theoretical notes, methodological notes, peer review notes, and general reflective notes.

6. A pattern appreciation profile is developed through a process of synopsis. A variety of methods may be used as long as these are consistent with the orientation of pattern appreciation and are shared with participant/respondent in informed consent.

7. The pattern appreciation profile is verified by the participant/respondent who has primary voice in the content and form of the profile. The scientist/practitioner has a facilitative role in the development of the profile.

8. A conceptual/theoretical synthesis is developed based on pattern information collected.

9. A peer review system may be created to assist the scientist/practitioner in assuring logical consistency of the process. It is desirable to engage a peer reviewer who is familiar with the conceptual system and the method. A peer reviewer's goal would be to enhance the reflective aspects of the process.

10. For the purposes of scientific credibility, audit procedures may be developed. These audit procedures would enable review of documentation for grounds of unitary knowledge claims of the participants. The auditor should be expert in unitary conceptual system and understand the method.

11. A case study report may be developed for publication or reporting to a funding source. This would include the pattern appreciation profile and the conceptual/theoretical synthesis. The participant/respondent has access to the pattern appreciation case report and may provide feedback for refinement of the report.

The critical elements of the pattern appreciation approach are outlined as a general guide for implementation. These elements should reflect the intent of the co-participants, the unfolding design of the overall endeavor and specific engagements, the creative expression of co-participants, and the negotiated positions of the co-participants. The unitary pattern appreciation approach is meant to be implemented within the context of the process, the orientation, and critical features specified.

CRITICAL FEATURES

There are three critical features of unitary pattern appreciation. Pattern appreciation is synoptic, participatory, and transformative. These features represent distinguishing hallmarks of this process, orientation, and approach.

Synoptic

The synoptic nature of pattern appreciation differentiates the process from analysis common to other forms of understanding information. It is consistent with a science of pandimensional unitary human beings. It is through synopsis that the full force or fullness of pattern is sought. Synopsis is the foundation for unitary knowing. Murphy (1992) used an approach for research on transformation developed by Broad (1953) as synoptic empiricism. "Synopsis is the deliberate viewing together of aspects of human experience which, for one reason or another, are generally kept apart by the plain man and even by the professional scientist or scholar. The object of synopsis is to try to find out how various aspects are inter-related" (p. 8). From a unitary perspective, the object of synopsis shifts away from the inter-relatedness of aspects because in a unitary view pattern manifestations reflect wholeness and integrality of human field. The object is not how data are inter-related, but "the clearest and fullest picture of unitary pattern that is reflected in data or information" (Cowling, 1993a, p. 206) arising in the pattern appreciation process. The pattern appreciation process is not seeking relatedness because integrality transcends relatedness. Pattern appreciation aims at compelling emergence of wholeness amidst the energetic manifestations of experience, perception, and expressions, the source of pattern information.

Synthesis flows from the process of synopsis. "Synthesis is the attempt to create a coherent set of concepts and principles which cover satisfactorily all the regions of fact which have been viewed synoptically" (Murphy, 1992, p. 8). In unitary pattern appreciation, synopsis is the grounding for a unitary conceptual/theoretical synthesis.

Participatory

The unitary pattern appreciation endeavor is a coparticipatory process throughout its conception and implementation. The scientist/practitioner and the participant/respondent in the endeavor have different but equally shared responsibility for the nature of the engagement and the unfolding process. While guidelines have been articulated in the previously described approach, all aspects of the endeavor are negotiated. The establishment of purpose, choice of methods for engagement, documentation, construction of a pattern profile, formulation of a conceptual/theoretical synthesis, and creation of case report are all co-paticipatory. In particular, the pattern appreciation profile format is dependent on the degree to which it captures and conveys the experience, perception, and expressions of the participant/respondent. Choices about language, form, and format of the profile are highly dependent on how meaningfully the profile portrays pattern from the participant/respondent's perspective.

The ideals of a participatory research/practice model inherent in unitary pattern appreciation are parallel to participatory research (Reason, 1988) and the practice model called Life Process System (Schaef, 1992). In the participatory or experiential research model, the researcher and respondents share control of the study through a collaborative process in all aspects of the inquiry process. The Life Process System model of practice advocates for practitioner receptivity to the client's life process. It also embraces honoring this process. The practitioner is not viewed as an intervener who interferes with the inherent healing capacity of the client. The client and practitioner are viewed as equal participants in any helping encounter. Knowledge is used as it arises from the experience of encounters and engagements. Theoretical knowledge is also derived from and used in encounters and engagements. Theory informs practice and practice informs theory. Participation in one's life process is at the heart of this model of practice. Surrender of practitioner control typical in helping relationships is a necessity of the life process model. This means giving up traditional notions of cause and effect which are central to control and intervention. Diagnosis is not the foundation for practice;

wisdom arising from participation with clients is the foundation. In its denial of the primacy of diagnosis, the model implies a rejection of a dualistic view of illness (ill and not-ill) and of judgment as a critical attribute for the potential of healing.

The participatory feature of pattern appreciation is a unitary reformulation using elements of participatory research and the life process model. This represents a creative synthesis of these two research and practice perspectives into a unitary science/practice model. In pattern appreciation, respondents are equal collaborators in the endeavor for understanding relevant to practice and science. Knowledge is developed in the context of the individual situation. The practitioner/scientist is receptive to and honoring of the patterning of the individual. The scientist/practitioner is not intervener or controller for purposes of practice or research. Unitary knowledge arises from the wisdom of the participation in appreciating pattern. Theoretical and practical knowledge arise simultaneously. The hallmark of unitary pattern appreciation is knowing participation in one's own patterning. The lack of causality and the unpredictable nature of change from a unitary perspective make control and intervention obsolete in this model. The referents for practice and science are unitary field pattern and pandimensionality. The participatory nature of unitary pattern appreciation is requisite to knowing participation in change which is a cornerstone of unitary thinking as espoused by Rogers (1992).

Transformative

The nature of unitary pattern appreciation is transformative. Within the perspective of the Science of Unitary Human Beings we are moving toward greater diversity, innovation, and complexity (Rogers, 1992). This movement and change occurs regardless of pattern appreciation. By asking participants to make pattern the referent of attention, unitary pattern appreciation creates a context for "new consciousness and enlightened awareness" of this unfolding stream of continuity. It replaces the attention on such aspects as age, the body, or the psychological state. Thus it is transformative.

Unitary pattern appreciation offers transformative potential in another way. It provides the context for not only making pattern referent for consciousness and awareness, it creates a context for making pandimensionality the referent for change. It asks participants to get in touch with the pandimensional nature of time, space, movement, and change. This process is very akin to the spiritual perspective of "unitive consciousness" or "the Second Miracle" described recently by Richard Moss (1995) in terms of a theory of evolution as growing complexity. To realize this consciousness is fundamental "is to become referent to infinity" (Moss, 1995, p. 62). The parallel in unitary pattern appreciation is to offer the possibility of becoming "referent to pandimensionality" because this unitary conceptualization of humans implies both infinite potential and infinite time-space-movement-change. The unitive consciousness, I believe, is the pandimensional consciousness. Moss (1995) describes it as: "an experience of realization that ends all referents by which to measure or categorize oneself or existence" (p. 63); "a deepening understanding of fundamental relationship between things that were formerly not seen as related" (p. 64); "in a great sea of being open in all directions to the infinite" (p. 65); "where feeling, sensation, and thinking are a unified continuum that is not limited to the boundaries of our body" (p. 65); "restores wholeness and connection" (p. 66); and "every moment is a new birth and what is being born is not merely the product of the past, not merely the cause of some earlier effect, but rather part of a ceaseless cosmos of revelation" (p. 66). If there is any clear goal of unitary pattern appreciation in relation to transformation, it would be as Moss (1995) sums it up: "To become referent to infinity is not to have our identity located in any finite notion of ourselves. We are movement and flow. Our careers, our health, our families, and possessions may temporarily represent a harbor for our sense of self, but ultimately we are always far more" (p. 67). The transformative quality of unitary pattern appreciation is reaching for this essence.

PARTING PERSPECTIVES

It is difficult to summarize the intent and meaning of unitary pattern appreciation. I have made so many discoveries in my search for an alternative approach to our traditional ways of doing the science and art of nursing that extends our rich traditions of service to human beings. One of those discoveries was the poet Gerard Manley Hopkins (Gardner, 1963: Roberts, 1994) and his concepts of *inscape* and *instress.* Inscape was the term he coined for "that individually distinctive form which constitutes the rich and revealing oneness of the natural object" (Gardner, 1963, p. xx). Instress was the term he used for "that energy of being by which all things are upheld" (p. xx). These two ideas are akin to the notions of pattern and energy inherent in Rogers' (1992) conceptualizations. Instress was conceptualized as the unifying force in the object and that which acts on the senses allowing perception by the beholder. "Instress, then, is often the *sensation* of inscape—a quasi-mystical illumination, a sudden perception of that deeper pattern, order, and unity which gives meaning to external forms" (Gardner, 1963, p. xxi). Roberts (1994) describes this as "an aesthetic experience where the emphasis is on the 'beauty' and pattern of what is seen; there is no attempt to analyze the why and how of these feelings" (p. 51). One of the virtues of inscape is its distinctiveness (Hopkins, as cited in Roberts, 1994, p. 34), much like the uniqueness of human field pattern. Gardner thinks that the mark of the artist is the feeling for this intrinsic quality and reaching for this pattern. Hopkins (as cited in Roberts, 1994) described it best himself, "so design, pattern, or what I am in the habit of calling 'inscape' is what I above all aim at in poetry" (p. 34). In unitary pattern appreciation the aim or mark of the artist (scientist/practitioner) is reaching for the essence of unitary pattern.

REFERENCES

Broad, C. D. (1953). *Religion, philosophy and psychical research.* New York: Harcourt, Brace.

Cowling, W. R. (1990). A template for unitary pattern-based nursing practice. In E. A. M. Barrett (Ed.), *Visions of Rogers' science-based nursing* (pp. 45-65). New York: NLN Press.

Cowling, W. R. (1993a). Unitary practice: Revisionary assumptions. In M. S. Parker (Ed.), *Nursing theories in practice* (Vol. 2). New York: NLN Press.

Cowling, W. R. (1993b). Unitary knowing in nursing practice. *Nursing Science Quarterly, 6,* 201-207.

Gardner, W. H. (1963). *Poems and prose of Gerard Manley Hopkins.* London: Penguin.

LeShan, L., & Margenau, H. (1982). *Einstein's space and Van Gogh's sky: Physical reality and beyond.* New York: Macmillan.

Moss, R. (1995). *The second miracle: Intimacy, spirituality, and conscious relationships.* Berkeley, CA: Celestial Arts.

Murphy, M. (1992). *The future of the body: Explorations into the further evolution of human nature.* Los Angeles: Tarcher.

The Oxford English dictionary (2nd ed.) [CD-ROM]. (1994). New York: Oxford University Press.

Reason, P. (Ed.). (1988). *Human inquiry in action: Developments in new paradigm research.* London: Sage.

Roberts, G. (1994). *Gerard Manley Hopkins: A literary life.* New York: St. Martin's.

Rogers, M. E. (1992). Nursing science and the space age. *Nursing Science Quarterly, 5,* 27-33.

Schaef, A. W. (1992). *Beyond therapy, beyond science.* New York: HarperCollins.

12

Pediatric Acquired Immunodeficiency Syndrome (AIDS) as Studied from a Rogerian Perspective: A Sense of Hope

Mary Ireland

*D*espite the significant reduction in mother-to-infant transmission of HIV and the improved health status of infants and children receiving zidovudine (protocol 076) (Connor et al., 1994), a cure for HIV remains elusive and HIV remains a threat for women and their children over the next decade (Gallagher & Klima, 1996). Although HIV disease in children is increasingly described as a chronic illness (Sherwen & Boland, 1994), its progression to AIDS, the final outcome, remains fatal.

Unfortunately, the accent of clinicians and researchers about fatally ill children, including those who are HIV-infected, has been on the psychopathological and defensive side of reactions to the process of fatal illness in children. This perspective fails to acknowledge that, as these children attempt to make meaning of the illness, they may advance to death and thereby come to terms with their mortality faster than their healthy peers.

Rogers stated (1988), "A new world view is necessary for a more productive approach to studying AIDS" (p. 101). Although pediatric AIDS is a fatal illness, it is more than a disease. It is a human event that requires a new perspective of existing knowledge about a child's development amid personal challenge, change, and transition.

ACCELERATING CHANGE THEORY:
AN ALTERNATIVE VIEW

The Science of Unitary Human Beings (Rogers, 1987) offers a model for perceiving people and gaining an understanding of the nature of the human life process. Individuals, viewed as unitary wholes, and different from the sum of their parts, are in mutual process with their environment. They are open systems living in a pandimensional universe of open systems, and described as energy fields identified by unique patterns. In the theory of accelerating change, Rogers (1986) suggests that change, which characterizes the human field pattern, may occur faster for some than for others. From this perspective, children who have AIDS may be seen as examples of rapidly changing field rhythms and their illness as an opportunity to advance their emotional growth. Adherents of a pandimensional perception of reality invalidate "chronological age as a basis for differentiating human change" (Rogers, 1992, p. 32). The development of AIDS-diagnosed children may be less associated with age, a linear time marker, and more with this life-changing event.

Rogers' (1986) principle of integrality identifies change as emerging from the environmental human field mutual process. Some developmental theorists hold the view that out of the infant-parent relationship, an early awareness of mortality emerges that antedates conceptual knowledge of death (Klein, 1948; Winnicott, 1960; Yalom, 1980). Maurer (1966) observed the young child's interest in disappearance and reappearance, and reasoned the infant's first task was to differentiate between self/not self, and thereby establish the distinction between being/nonbeing, life and death.

The principle of helicy specifies increasing diversity of field patterns (See Appendix). Although a rudimentary conceptualization of death evolves via periods of separation from the caretaker and death-related games and conversation (Katzenbaum, 1977), there is accumulating evidence that experience with death, such as the death of a family member, may facilitate a more mature awareness of death in children, regardless of age and cognitive level (Cotton & Range, 1990; Kane, 1979; Reilly, Hasazi, & Bond, 1983; Schonfeld & Smilansky, 1989), especially during the subjectively relevant event of fatal illness (Bearison & Pacifici, 1984; Bluebond-Langner, 1975, 1989; Goodman, 1989, Kübler-Ross, 1974). According to Spinetta and Deasy-Spinetta (1981), the fatally ill child tries to make meaning out of an emotionally charged environment and, in the process, may become aware of his or her impending death earlier than healthy peers.

The nature of change experienced by both fatally ill and healthy children is underwritten in Rogers' (1986) Science of Unitary Human Beings and is made manifest in the theory of accelerating change. The life experiences of fatally ill children evidence this acceleration. Taking medications, hospitalization, clinic visits, experiencing pain, and the death of peers all advance illness-related knowledge. Fatally ill children recognize that adult caretakers treat them differently. By combining information about people's behaviors with tests and treatments received, these children rapidly comprehend that they are seriously ill (Bluebond-Langner, 1975). They have been described as advanced beyond their years (Bearison & Pacifici, 1984; Kübler-Ross, 1974) and reported, on occasion, to have images and sensations that convey acceleration, for example, "travelling on a very fast train" or "free falling in outerspace" (Fagen, 1982, p. 19). Lipson (1993) said that "in such an unpredictable disease as pediatric AIDS, some children obtain a precocious grasp of life-and-death issues" (p. 9).

Human beings manifest increasing diversity, and appear to thrive on change (Rogers, 1990). Although Halpern and Palic (1984) reported death anxiety present in children as early as ages three to four years, Koocher, O'Malley, Gogan, and Foster (1976) suggested that age alone was not a factor from which to predict the degree of death anxiety in children, but that life experiences might be important determinants. Maddi (1980) wrote that confrontation with and acknowledgment of the imminence of one's death can sensitize an individual to the meaningfulness of life, and thereby reduce anxiety. Goodman (1989) reported that, while children with cancer were aware that their illness could be fatal, this knowledge was not associated with increased anxiety. Similarly, Hagey (1990) reported that terminally ill children 5 to 12 years of age did not have greater death concern than the chronically ill or healthy control groups studied. He said, "This trend is exactly counter" (p. 191) to what was found in the literature about ill children. It is possible that the intensified awareness of life's transience experienced by the fatally ill child who has AIDS may advance personal growth and pave the way for decreased death anxiety.

Rogers (1987, 1990) provides a model that perceives self-awareness emerging out of the mutual human-environmental process; that is, the personal construction of one's reality occurs early in life and involves action of self with others. Most self-esteem theorists acknowledge that this human attribute develops through the experiencing of the parent (Coopersmith, 1967; Harter, 1990). There is now evidence of early self-evaluative abilities in preschool children (Anderson & Adams, 1985; Stipek & Hoffman, 1980) and that the environment plays a role in producing these skills (Harter, 1990). Self-affirmation and the foundation for the degree to which the child holds self-worth and value enfolds through the human/environmental field mutual process. The child's experiencing of the parent early in life is focal in this human/environmental process.

According to Rogers (1986), "More diverse field patterns change more rapidly than less diverse" (p. 7). Harter (1987) wrote that self-esteem in the young child is viewed as a sense of adequacy in the dimensions of competence and social acceptance, and that conflict may facilitate the transition from an all-or-nothing to a more mature appraisal of self-feelings. According to B. Sourkes, a child psychologist, who for 15 years has worked with children who have cancer, fatal illness pushes the child to a nonage-related kind of awareness, wherein self-feelings become age-less (personal communication, October 4, 1993). Morse (1990) reported that children ages 3 to 16 years who survived critical illness and Near Death Experience (NDE) showed more realistic self-appraisals and self-confidence after experiencing these events. From this perspective, fatal illness can be viewed as an experience that changes the child's life and heightens self-awareness (Bluebond-Langner, 1975; Sourkes, 1991). Increased awareness sets the stage for new self-learning with the possibility of experiencing an enhancement of self-esteem in children with AIDS.

IN THEIR OWN VOICE:
CHILDREN WITH AIDS SPEAK OUT

Using the theory of accelerating change, the author conducted a descriptive study that examined differences in two human field manifestations, death anxiety and self-esteem in African-American and Latino healthy and AIDS-diagnosed children, four, five, and six years of age. It was hypothesized that children who have AIDS would manifest lower death anxiety and higher self-esteem than minority children who are healthy.

To develop a death anxiety profile, children were administered the projective instrument, Thematic Instrument for Measuring Death Anxiety in Children (TIMDAC) (Ireland, 1994). Responses children made to four chromatic pictures, a subset taken from 23 plates developed for Tell-Me-A-Story (TEMAS) (Costantino, Malgady, & Rogler. 1988), were scored. These pictures were chosen since they were found to elicit themes of death and death anxiety when shown to children. The stories told by children who had AIDS did not express more themes of death anxiety than their healthy peers. In particular, their stories had fewer death-related themes of being abandoned or separated from significant figures or having feelings of sadness or fear about being abandoned or separated from these figures.

For example, a little girl with AIDS told the following story about a picture of a child standing in a forest before a large, dark tree. There was a path with people to the right of the tree and to the left, an empty path. "The girl touched the tree and fell down, crying and crying. The father said hi, little girl I love you. And then the tree is alive like a monster, and the monster took her away. But the father cuts the tree monster—chock, chock—and the monster is gone and then the girl is safe." Another AIDS-diagnosed child, viewing the same picture, said that the child in front of the tree was praying and the little people on the path were praying with the child. The first child expressed a threatening situation, but she does not feel abandoned. On the contrary, the father successfully rescues her. Interestingly, the second child conveys a strong sense of communion with others. B. Sourkes (1991), spoke of a kind of spiritual inwardness she has observed in children who have cancer.

Lamendola and Newman (1994) reported that, following cycles of aloneness and searching, some adult HIV-infected and AIDS-diagnosed adults reached a turning point, a juncture that the authors described as a "unitary-transformative experience" (p. 20). Not unlike these adults, for the AIDS-diagnosed children, it would appear that the meaning of fatal illness was evolving as an accelerated awareness of the living-dying experience and as a manifestation of higher frequency field patterning. If fatally ill children are able to transcend themselves, they may think less about being separated from, or being abandoned by loved ones and become more concerned about the well-being of those they will leave behind when they die.

The author observed very close attachments, that is, the human/environmental mutual process was intense with a focus on the AIDS-diagnosed children and their caretakers. This process appeared even more accelerated when the caretaker was a biological mother who was HIV-infected.

To explore manifestations of self-esteem, the Pictorial Scale of Perceived Competence and Social Acceptance (PSCA) (Harter & Pike, 1984), a 24-picture and item instrument that measures a child's sense of worth in the areas of perceived competence and social acceptance, was administered. Child self-esteem scores were obtained by asking a child to point to the child most like him or her in each of the 24 pictures.

Overall, the AIDS-diagnosed children were not discernably different from healthy peers in self-esteem. They did, however, perceive themselves as less cognitively competent. Their lower scores in self-evaluation of cognitive competence should be examined in light of the fact that our knowledge about the cognitive abilities of children with HIV/AIDS is less than comprehensive and complete and has been heavily dominated with discussions of neurological and developmental defects. Although high rates of neurodevelopmental involvement and cognitive delays have been reported about children with AIDS (Diamond, Wiznia, Belman, Rubenstein, & Cohen, 1990), study design flaws (Armstrong, Seidel, & Swales, 1993), small sample sizes, use of different tools to assess cognitive functioning, and a focus on infant development (Levenson, Mellins, Zawadzki, Kairam, & Stein, 1992) have complicated interpretation of findings. Despite the fact that some of the AIDS-diagnosed children had language and cognitive impairments, all expressed feelings about self-worth. Some, by the nature of their experiences, for example, loss of developmental milestones, provided a more realistic appraisal of themselves and their abilities. As one child said in response to a picture of two children, one of whom is reported to be very good at numbers and the other, just pretty good, "I'm not so good at counting." It is possible that their honest self-appraisals of cognitive competence contributed to the significantly lower scores on this subscale, conveying an honesty seldom seen with self-reports by either adults or children.

Rogers (1994) stated, "We are in the midst of a rapid shift from the traditional world view, an old reality. We are living in the midst of a new reality that is already transcending what we have long taken for granted" (p. 33). In this study, the manifestations of death anxiety and self-esteem in children 4, 5, and 6 years of age who have AIDS were not significantly different than their healthy peers. These findings contradict the conventional perspective that fatally ill children are, by and large, emotionally dysfunctional and provide a different view about children who have fatal illnesses. They may possess a strength overlooked previously.

A SENSE OF HOPE

These results convey a sense of hope in contrast to the prevailing view of despair and gloom that has surrounded the stigma, guilt, and tragedy of pediatric AIDS. A picture of the AIDS-diagnosed children, characterized as being far more than the passive victims we have assumed them to be, was made manifest using Rogers' nursing model as a theoretic source of knowledge. Using Rogers' visionary model offered an opportunity to challenge some of the shibboleths about ways of knowing and understanding children who have fatal illness. There is no single, exclusive way of describing their reality, and these, the "youngest heroes," have helped to illuminate and clarify how the world is for them. Having established in some measure, that, in the face of adversity, children can achieve higher levels of being holds out promise to a world struggling to bring meaning not only to pediatric AIDS, but other current dilemmas as well. From this perspective, the nurse cannot participate only in the fatally ill child's transformative experience, but can facilitate the child's ability to extract meaning from it. To help a child complete this journey requires a commitment toward hope and staying focused on that which is central to nursing, the betterment of humankind.

M. E. Rogers (1994) wrote, "I happen to believe that people need knowledgeable nursing. . . . "(p. 35). As nurses caring for persons with AIDS, we have an opportunity and responsibility to direct new ways of thinking about the meaning of life's living-dying rhythms.

REFERENCES

Anderson, P. L., & Adams, P. J. (1985). The relationship of five-year-olds' academic readiness and perceptions of competence and acceptance. *Journal of Educational Psychology, 79*(2), 114-118.

Armstrong, F. D., Seidel, J. F., & Swales, T. P. (1993). Pediatric HIV infection: A neuropsychological and educational challenge. *Journal of Learning Disabilities, 26*(2), 92-103.

Bearison, D., & Pacifici, R. (1984). Psychological studies of children who have cancer. *Journal of Applied Developmental Psychology, 10,* 469-486.

Bluebond-Langner, M. (1975). *Awareness and communication in terminally ill children: Pattern, process, and pretense.* Unpublished doctoral dissertation, University of Illinois, Urbana-Champaign.

Bluebond-Langner, M. (1989). Worlds of dying children and their well siblings. *Death Studies, 13,*1-16.

Connor, E., Sperling, R., Gelber, R., Kiselev, P., Scott, G., O'Sullivan, M., VanDyke, R., Mohammed, B., Shearer, W., Jacobson, M., Jemenez, E., O'Neill, E., Bazin, B., Delfraissy, J., Culnane, M., Coombs, R., Elkins, M., Moye, J., Stratton, P., & Balsley J. (1994). Reduction of maternal-infant transmission of human immunodeficiency virus type I with zidovudine treatment. *New England Journal of Medicine, 331*(11), 1173-1180.

Coopersmith, S. (1967). *The antecedents of self-esteem.* Palo Alto: Consulting Psychologist Press.

Costantino, G., Malgady, R., & Rogler, L. (1988). *TEMAS (Tell-Me-A-Story) manual*. Los Angeles: Western Psychological Services.

Cotton, C. R., & Range, L. M. (1990). Children's death concepts: Relationship to cognitive functioning, age, experience with death, fear of death, and hopelessness. *Journal of Clinical Child Psychology, 19*(2), 123–127.

Diamond, G. W., Wiznia, A. A., Belman, A. L., Rubenstein, A., & Cohen, H. L. (1990). Effects of congenital HIV infection on neurodevelopmental status in foster care. *Developmental Medicine and Child Neurology, 32*, 999–1005.

Fagen, T. S. (1982). Music therapy in the treatment of anxiety and fear in terminal pediatric patients. *Music Therapy, 2*, 13–23.

Gallagher, M. A., & Klima, C. (1996). The challenge of maternal-infant transmission of HIV. *Journal of the Association of Nurses in AIDS Care, 7*(1), 47–48.

Goodman, R. F. (1989). *Development of the concept of death in children: The cognitive and affective components*. Unpublished doctoral dissertation, Adelphi University, New York.

Hagey, E. M. (1990). A developmental study of terminally-ill, chronically-ill and physically healthy children's concerns with and cognitive evaluation of death. *Dissertation Abstracts International, 54*(01), (University Microfilms No. 91-05,561)

Halpern, E., & Palic, L. (1984). Developmental changes in death anxiety in childhood. *Journal of Applied Developmental Psychology, 5*, 163–172.

Harter, S. (1987). The determinants and mediational role of global self-worth in children. In N. Eisenberg (Ed.), *Contemporary topics in developmental psychology* (pp. 219–242). New York: John Wiley & Sons.

Harter, S. (1990). Causes, correlates, and the functional role of global self-worth. In J. Kolligian & R. Sternberg (Eds.), *Perceptions of competence and incompetence across the life-span* (pp. 67–100). New Haven, CT: Yale University.

Harter, S., & Pike, R. (1984). The pictorial scale of perceived competence and social acceptance for young children. *Child Development, 55*, 1969–1982.

Ireland, M. (1994). *Death anxiety and self-esteem in children four, five and six years of age: A comparison of minority children who have AIDS with minority children who are healthy*. Unpublished doctoral dissertation, New York University, New York.

Kane, B. (1979). Children's concepts of death. *The Journal of Genetic Psychology, 134*, 141–153.

Katzenbaum, R. J. (1977). *Death, society, and human experience*. St. Louis, MO: Mosby.

Klein, M. (1948). A contribution to the theory of anxiety and guilt. *International Journal of Psychoanalysis, 29*, 114–123.

Koocher, G. P., O'Malley, J. E., Gogan, J. L., & Foster, D. J. (1976). Psychological adjustment among pediatric cancer survivors. *Journal of Child Psychology and Psychiatry, 21*, 163–173.

Kübler-Ross, E. (1974). Thanatos: Disease. *Journal of Clinical Psychology, 3*, 22–24.

Lamendola, F. P., & Newman, M. A. (1994). The paradox of HIV/AIDS as expanding consciousness. *Advances in Nursing Science, 16*(3), 13–21.

Levenson, R. L., Mellins, C. A., Zawadzki, M., Kairam, & Stein, Z. (1992). Cognitive assessment of human immunodeficiency virus-exposed children. *American Journal of Diseases of Children, 146,* 1479-1483.

Lipson, M. (1993). What do you say to the child with AIDS? *Hastings Center Report, 23*(2), 6-12.

Maddi, S., (1980). Developmental value of fear of death. *The Journal of Mind and Behavior, 1*(1), 85-92.

Maurer, A. (1966). Maturation concepts of death. *British Journal of Medical Psychology, 39*(35), 35-41.

Morse, M. (1990). *Closer to the light.* New York: Villard Books.

Reilly, T. P., Hasazi, J. E., & Bond, L. A. (1983). Children's conceptions of death and personal mortality. *Journal of Pediatric Psychology, 8*(1), 21-31.

Rogers, M. E. (1986). Science of unitary human beings. In V. M. Malenski (Ed.), *Explorations on Martha Rogers' science of unitary human beings* (pp. 3-8). Norwalk, CT: Appleton-Century-Crofts.

Rogers, M. E. (1987). Rogers' science of unitary human beings. In R. R. Parse (Ed.), *Nursing science: Major paradigms, theories, and critiques* (pp. 139-146). Philadelphia: W. B. Saunders.

Rogers, M. E. (1988). Nursing science and art: A prospective. *Nursing Science Quarterly, 1,* 99-102.

Rogers, M. E. (1990). Nursing: Science of unitary, irreducible, human beings: Update 1990. In E. A. M. Barrett (Ed.), *Visions of Rogers' science-based nursing* (pp. 5-11). New York: NLN Press.

Rogers, M. E. (1992). Nursing science and the space age. *Nursing Science Quarterly, 5,* 27-34.

Rogers, M. E. (1994). The science of unitary human beings: Current perspectives. *Nursing Science Quarterly, 7,* 33-35.

Schonfeld, D. J., & Smilansky, S. (1989). A cross-cultural comparison of Israeli and American children's death concepts. *Death Studies, 13,* 593-604.

Sherwen, L. N., & Boland, M. (1994). Overview of psychosocial research concerning pediatric human immunodeficiency virus infection. *Developmental and Behavioral Pediatrics, 15*(Suppl. 3), 5-11.

Sourkes, B. M. (1991). *The deepening shade: Psychological aspects of life-threatening illness.* Pittsburgh, PA: Pittsburgh Press.

Spinetta, J. J., & Deasy-Spinetta, P. (1981). Talking with children who have a life-threatening illness. In J. J. Spinetta & P. Deasy-Spinetta (Eds.), *Living with childhood cancer* (pp.234-252).

Stipek, D. J., & Hoffman, J. M. (1980). Development of children's performance-related judgements. *Child Development, 51,* 912-914.

Winnicott, D. W. (1960). The theory of the parent-infant relationship. *International Journal of Psychoanalysis, 41,* 585-595.

Yalom, I. (1980). *Existential psychotherapy.* New York: Basic Books.

13

Well-Being and High-Risk Drug Use Among Active Drug Users

*Marcia Andersen and
Elaine M. Hockman*

During a three-year period, a group of nurses and outreach workers in Detroit, Michigan, provided healthcare services to two groups of active heroin and cocaine users. These healthcare services were designed to assist in the reduction of risk of contracting AIDS. Both study groups received HIV testing, pre- and post-HIV education/counseling sessions, and HIV blood tests. In addition, one group, randomized by recruitment zip code, participated in the Personalized Nursing LIGHT Practice Model Intervention—a practice model of the art of nursing based on Martha Rogers' Science of Unitary Human Beings (Andersen & Smereck, 1989, 1992; Andersen, Smereck, & Hockman, 1996). The goal of the LIGHT Model is to assist clients in improving their sense of well-being, thus enabling them to perceive wider varieties of options and possible actions in

152

their lives. We also postulated that such perception would be associated with a higher probability of selecting behaviors "less risky" to health from previous behaviors.

In this chapter, we describe a pre-post research study involving a correlational design to determine if there is a relationship between change in well-being and change in high-risk drug-related behaviors related to AIDS acquisition and transmission. Analysis showed that improvement of active drug users' sense of well-being was associated with being in the presence of nurses and nursing support staff who practiced the Personalized Nursing LIGHT Model. Furthermore, an improved sense of well-being was associated with a decrease in high-risk AIDS-related behaviors.

STUDY METHODS

Purpose

The overarching premise of this study was that exposure to an educational program would be associated with subjects' reducing the extent to which they engage in behaviors that put them at risk for contracting HIV. Furthermore, there should be additional reductions in risk behavior for subjects who receive additional treatment—in this case, participation in the Rogerian-based Personalized Nursing LIGHT practice model of nursing.

Theoretical Framework and Treatment Groups

Standard Care.   The standard education/counseling program (consisting of two sessions) was attended by all participants and was conducted by outreach workers who were recovering indigenous staff, trained in HIV counseling. The standard program protocol was based on several theories of behavior change, including the Social Influence Theory, Health Belief Model, Fear Arousal Theory, and Social Learning Theory. A manual for the standard program procedures, prepared by Susan Coyle at the National Institute on Drug Abuse (Coyle, 1993), consisted of two teaching/counseling sessions encompassing HIV and antibody screening. The program was designed to be culturally appropriate to the high-risk lifestyle of the active male or female drug user.

During the teaching/counseling sessions, cue cards were used to assure strict adherence to the standard protocol. The first session concentrated on HIV pre-test counseling. Clients were educated about what HIV is, how testing is done, and the potential outcomes. Secondary purposes of the first visit were to teach appropriate risk-reduction strategies and demonstrate necessary skills for properly cleaning needles and putting on a condom. After this 20–30 minute visit, if the client wished, confidential and private HIV testing was conducted at a nearby testing laboratory.

Two or three weeks later the client returned for a second session whose content varied, depending on whether the client was HIV positive or negative or had not been tested. This session was a "booster" session for HIV negative clients and clients who declined testing. The second session, which took approximately 20–40 minutes, provided the following information:

- HIV test result, if applicable,
- The meaning of HIV positive and negative results and discussion of risk reduction,
- Review of HIV prevention strategies,
- Distribution of HIV literature and HIV service referrals, and
- Distribution of social and economic service referrals.

The second session took longer (40–60 minutes) for HIV positive subjects. Clients who tested seropositive received their test results and then discussed with a staff member the meaning of the results, including medical follow-up and early treatment options as well as receiving HIV/AIDS literature and referral information. This discussion was based on a set of three cue cards (Coyle, 1993). All subjects were asked to return in approximately six months for follow-up appraisal.

LIGHT: The Enhanced Care. After participating in the standard care provided, approximately half the subjects, drawn from randomly selected zip codes, were assigned to additional enhanced care—the LIGHT Model as based on Rogers' Science of Nursing (Andersen, 1986; Andersen & Smereck, 1989, 1992) and as used effectively in previous studies (Andersen & Braunstein, 1992; Andersen, Smereck, & Braunstein, 1993). Turn to the discussion section for a more detailed description of how the LIGHT Model was integrated within the present study.

Subject Recruitment and Initial Procedures

Regions of Detroit, identified by secondary sources as being high drug-use areas, were mapped to determine the probable density of drug use and AIDS risk in a prescribed geographic area (Braunstein, 1993). Four postal code zones, two for each study group, were selected. Police, health department officials, and individuals in drug treatment programs confirmed these as high drug-use areas. Street-by-street observation verified the study sites. Recruitment occurred within these zip code areas with no residence requirement, though the individuals often lived there. Two of the zip code areas accounted for the residence of 72.1 percent of the standard subjects (44.1% in one area and 28% in another); one zip code accounted for 72.9 percent of the subjects who received the enhanced treatment. Part way through the study, the zip codes were switched —the LIGHT zip codes became standard treatment areas and the "standard" zip codes became the LIGHT areas.

Recruitment of clients was achieved by ethnically matching outreach workers to the communities in which they worked. The outreach workers went to areas known to have a high frequency of drug use and drug "copping." (Copping means the drug user is picking up the drug from one place and taking it elsewhere to use.)

Men and women eligible for inclusion in the study were: 18 years or older, self-identified as an injecting drug user or crack cocaine user within the last 48 hours, and agreeable to confirmation by a urine test, medically stable, and not currently enrolled in any long-term drug treatment program.

Once the subject gave informed consent to participate in the study, he or she was driven by van to the community office where drug use within the last 48 hours was confirmed via a urine test.

Roche Ontrak urine tests were used on site. To ensure accurate urine drug test results, the office staff used an "eyeball to meatus—chain of custody" method to administer the test, never taking their eyes off the urine sample from collection until testing was completed for cocaine and/or heroin use.

Data Collection Instruments

Data collection instruments used in this phase were: The Risk Behavior Assessment (RBA) and a follow-up version, the Risk Behavior Follow-Up Assessment (RBFA), the Global Well-Being Index, and the Addiction Severity Index (ASI). The RBA and RBFA were used to assess baseline and follow-up demographic information, drug usage behaviors (both past and present), sexual practices, health status, and AIDS-related knowledge. Several recent studies report that respondents, when tested with these instruments, consistently and accurately reported drug use, injecting behaviors, and sexual practices (Dowling-Guyer et al., 1994; Needle et al.,1995; Weatherby et al., 1994).

The Global Well-Being Index, administered at both baseline and follow-up testing, measured each client's sense of well-being. Theoretically, well-being is defined as the maximum use of one's talents toward self-actualization (Aristotle, 1984) within one's potential (Rogers, 1986). Life satisfaction to date operationalizes the concept. Using an index of global well-being developed by Andrews and Withey (1976), nurses asked clients to describe how they felt about their lives as a whole on a seven-point scale ranging from "terrible" to "delighted." Nurses probed and asked clients why they answered as they did to develop a valid plan to assist the clients to improve well-being. In addition to the life satisfaction item, which was asked twice during the session, 19 questions, asking about specific areas of the client's life, were asked to enhance information on areas of life satisfaction clients believed could use improvement. Test-retest reliability coefficients from four national surveys ranged from .61 to .71 (Andrews & Withey, 1976).

The ASI, developed by McLellan et al. (1985), assessed seven areas of functioning often found to be impaired in drug-dependent individuals such as medical, legal, psychiatric, and employment/support status, family relationships, social relationships, and drugs/alcohol problems. The first six areas of the ASI were used at both baseline and follow-up. The drugs/alcohol items were omitted because of overlap with RBA and RBFA content. Addiction severity in each of the six areas was measured by summing the ratings given to troublesomeness of the problem and to the importance of getting help for it. In the literature, the reliability and validity of the ASI were initially tested twice on veteran populations with satisfactory results by the developers and have been verified in three drug treatment programs. Interrater reliability among interviewers, test-retest reliability, and validity were assessed. The correlations among eight interviewers ranged from .71 to .91, indicating satisfactory interrater reliability. There were no significant differences on any of the scales on a test-retest assessment (three days apart). Satisfactory correlation between the ASI functional scales and valid measures of each area, except for legal status, were found in a study of 181 patients. No satisfactory concurrent measure of legal status was identified (McLellan et al., 1985).

The Subjects

Subjects (N=744) were recruited over a three-year period; by design 70 percent were males; 30 percent females. Three hundred seventy-five (375) received standard care and three hundred sixty-nine (369) received LIGHT Model care in addition to standard care.

Retention and Follow-Up. Due to the diligent efforts of our outreach workers, the project enjoyed a 72 percent follow-up rate. A total of 454 subjects, or 61 percent of the initial recruits, had complete data from baseline and follow-up assessments and provided the sample for the analysis in this paper. The drug population was transient so it was often difficult to locate clients for their return visits. One of the outreach workers explained, "Calendars and clocks don't mean anything to many of these people." The second interview was done as close to six months after the initial interview as possible. The time span ranged from five to nine months.

ANALYSIS

The first order of analysis was to answer the question, "Did subjects, regardless of treatment type, decrease their risk behaviors?" The answer was a resounding, "Yes." (Hockman, 1994; Personalized Nursing Corporation, 1995). However, the question of greatest importance to our research was whether risk reduction was related to improvement in sense of well-being.

We needed to determine (a) whether the LIGHT subjects improved (reduced risk behavior) above and beyond the improvement (reduction) expected due to participation in the standard treatment and (b) whether this additional improvement was related to improvement in well-being. Analysis was complicated since there was no control group and both groups received the same standard care. A regression model was therefore used to determine the relationship between baseline and follow-up measures in the standard treatment group. The constants of these equations were applied to the measures from the LIGHT treatment group. The residuals (differences between their actual measured follow-up responses and their predicted follow-up responses based upon what would be expected due to participation in the standard treatment alone) were computed and used as our outcome variables to test the association between improvement in well-being and reduction in risk behaviors.

Aggregation of Well-Being Measures

The baseline responses to the well-being instrument were factor-analyzed to construct reliable scales. The procedures used for these data reductions are detailed in Personalized Nursing Corporation's Final Report (Hockman, 1994; Personalized Nursing Corporation, 1995). The factor analysis resulted in four meaningful factors, for which unweighted summative scores were computed at both baseline and follow-up. The first factor reflected a general satisfaction with one's life. Baseline reliability was .83; follow-up

.87. The second factor dealt with satisfaction with interpersonal relation-ships. Baseline reliability was .76; follow-up .79. The third factor repre-sented satisfaction with one's economic condition. Baseline reliability was .81; follow-up .86. The fourth factor dealt with satisfaction with one's com-munity. Baseline reliability was .85; follow-up .86.

Factor Analysis of the Aggregated Measures

Both at baseline and follow-up, six aggregate status measures were de-rived from the ASI—medical, legal, employment/support, psychiatric, family, and social; four satisfaction measures were derived from the well-being inventory—general, interpersonal relationships, one's economic condition, and one's community. Four drug usage variables were derived from the RBA/RBFA, and four measures of sex-related behaviors were de-rived from the RBA/RBFA.

The 18 aggregate baseline measures were factor analyzed, and corre-sponding baseline factor scores were computed to serve as composite measures. Five meaningful factors found at baseline, accounted for 61 percent of the variance. These factors mapped very well to the four areas under study; drug usage, sexual practice, well-being, and addiction sever-ity. Addiction severity measures loaded on two orthogonal factors repre-senting: (a) personal, or internal, aspects of concern (psychological, social, and family) and (b) aspects of concern that involve use of external systems (employment, legal, and medical care). The drug usage factor dealt mainly with injection practices.

The same set of 18 measures, derived from the RBFA, were also factor analyzed. Six meaningful factors accounted for 66 percent of the variance. The two addiction severity factors and well-being factor were duplicated in the follow-up factor solution. Two factors clearly represented (a) drug injection and (b) sexual practices. The sixth factor included crack use and the number of sex partners. Six follow-up factor scores were computed.

In summary, all of these factor scores at baseline and follow-up repre-sent aggregated scores to facilitate comparison. For all factor scores com-puted, a high score represents the undesirable behavior or feeling. The factor scores are on a z-score scale, with grand mean of zero and standard deviation of 1 in the total sample used for each factor analysis. The com-plete factor analyses for both baseline and follow-up data are presented in Personalized Nursing Corporation (1995).

Regression Results

The changes in risk associated with changes in well-being were based on two factors. First; simple linear regression was used to predict follow-up

factor scores from the corresponding baseline factor scores (e.g., baseline well-being factor score, predicting follow-up well-being factor
score) in the standard treatment sample. The equations derived from
this step were applied to the baseline factor scores for the LIGHT sample. Residual scores were computed for the LIGHT subjects. These residuals can be used as surrogates of change measures (i.e., as measures of
change in risk behavior and as measures of change in well-being and addiction severity). Basically, these residuals tell whether subjects are
doing as expected, better than expected, or worse than expected, had
they experienced standard care alone.

Second, multiple regression was used within the LIGHT subjects to predict risk behavior residuals from the well-being and addiction severity
residuals. Residuals are, as previously defined, the difference between actual (or obtained) value and predicted value. The equation is:

$$\text{Residual} = \text{Actual value} - \text{Predicted value}$$

The rationale for this analysis is that the premise being tested deals
with change:

• Improving well-being reduces risk
• Reducing addiction severity reduces risk.

Residuals reflect deviation from the expected and thus are considered
a measure of change.

• Did the client improve more than expected? or
• Did the client improve less than expected?

As the factor (construct) scores have been derived, high scores are
equated with high-risk, lack of well-being, or severe addiction problem:

• Negative residuals indicate improvement, and
• Positive residuals indicate worsening.

Therefore, in the multiple regression as a test of the theory, a positive
beta indicates an improvement in the well-being variable (independent
variable) and is associated with an improvement in risk behavior (dependent variable). Results by year end for the total LIGHT subjects are presented in Table 13.1; for standard subjects, in Table 13.2. For the LIGHT
subjects, the multiple correlation, R, was .30 (p=.0001); while for the
standard subjects, R=.12 (p=.3254).

Table 13.1   Change in Injection Risk as Function of Change in Well-Being: Light Treatment Subjects

Predictive Measures	N	Entry Year	Beta	t
General well-being	72	1992	.17	1.51
	97	1993	.23	2.34*
	52	1994	.38	2.66*
ASI: Internal aspects	72	1992	.33	2.87*
(psychological, social, & family	97	1993	−.08	.85
concerns)	52	1994	.07	.51
ASI: Aspects that involve use	72	1992	−.12	1.07
of external systems (employ-	97	1993	−.15	1.50
ment, legal, & medical concerns)	52	1994	−.06	.42
General well-being	221	all	.238	3.66*
ASI: Internal aspects			.168	2.58*
ASI: Aspects that involve use			−.096	1.48*
of external systems				

$^*p < .05$; Signs of betas are all in hypothesized direction.

Table 13.2   Change in Injection Risk as Function of Change in Well-Being: Standard Treatment Subjects

Predictive Measures	N	Entry Year	Beta	t
General well-being	66	1992	−.10	.82
	86	1993	−.01	.09
	81	1994	−.13	1.19
ASI: Internal aspects	66	1992	−.04	.30
(psychological, social, & family	86	1993	.02	.22
concerns)	81	1994	.01	.07
ASI: Aspects that involve use	66	1992	−.14	1.06
of external systems (employ-	86	1993	−.12	1.07
ment, legal, & medical concerns)	81	1994	−.276	2.42*
General well-being	233	all	−.07	1.01
ASI: Internal aspects			−.01	.13
ASI: Aspects that involve use			−.11	1.61
of external systems				

$^*p < .05$; However, the sign of the beta is in the opposite direction to that expected.

In the enhanced sample, the multiple regression equation to predict residuals on drug injection risk behavior was significant and the beta weights for well-being and psychological addiction severity were both significant. There were no significant results for the standard sample with respect to well-being and addiction severity. The hypotheses that improvement in well-being and reduction of addiction severity, as a result of participation in the LIGHT Model, leads to further reduction in risk behaviors was supported.

DISCUSSION

Findings

For the first year of LIGHT Model subjects, improvement with respect to internal concerns was significantly associated with reduction in injection risk behavior. As well-being and internal aspects of addiction severity (psychological, social, and family concerns) improved, risk behavior was reduced. In years two and three, improvement in well-being was significantly associated with reduction in injection risk behavior. For the entire LIGHT Model sample, both improvement in well-being and reduction in internal concerns were significantly associated with reduction in injection risk behaviors.

For the standard treatment subjects, there was only one significant association; an *increase* in external concerns (employment, legal, and medical) was associated with a decrease in injection risk behavior for third-year standard subjects. For the most part, however, well-being was unrelated to risk behavior for the standard subjects.

We must now look at what makes up the LIGHT treatment.

The Personalized Nursing LIGHT Practice Model: What Is It?

The LIGHT subjects experienced the Personalized Nursing LIGHT Practice Model, a model of the art of nursing based on the Science of Unitary Human Beings (Andersen & Smereck, 1989, 1992; Andersen, Smereck, & Braunstein, 1993). The practice model describes a process for deliberate change designed to improve well-being.

Two Phases of the Process for Nurses Practicing Within the Rogerian Science of Nursing.   Barrett (1990) states that, "The Rogerian practice methodology (Barrett, 1988) calls for (1) pattern manifestation appraisal and (2) deliberative mutual patterning. The nurse and client . . . work together to facilitate well-being throughout the life process" (p. 33).

Pattern Appraisal. Barrett (1990) defines pattern manifestation appraisal as "the continuous process of identifying manifestations of the human and environmental fields that relate to current health events. In practice the nurse identifies manifestations of pattern of both the client's human field and environmental field, recognizing the integral nature of the two fields" (p. 33).

A pattern is a distinguishing characteristic of an energy field (Rogers, 1990). Choices lead to certain distinguishing characteristics of energy fields or patterns.

Pattern Appraisal Process. The Personalized Nursing practice model uses a teaching heuristic called the Rainbow of Awareness to name pattern manifestations (Andersen & Smereck, 1994). This helps clients identify the patterns and frequencies of the energy patterns they manifest. These patterns are based on choices they make in their everyday lives.

Colors on the rainbow are used to depict increasingly higher frequency behavior patterns. Since the colors blue and purple have higher energy frequencies than the colors red and orange, we use blue and purple to represent the highest frequency human energy patterns associated with choices, behaviors, and attitudes.

Once clients identify the choices they usually make when confronted with experiences in the moment, they have a heightened awareness and more diverse field patterns emerge through the human environmental mutual process.

In order to facilitate knowing pattern change, it is important the clients understand and do pattern appraisal for themselves.

Facets of the Pattern Appraisal Process Using the Rainbow of Awareness

1. Ask the clients to name a painful experience.
2. Encourage them to "be in the moment" in a safe place with the experience/feeling.
3. Help them identify the choices they usually make during experiences like the one they named.
4. Help them identify pattern manifestations associated with their usual choices.

Deliberative Mutual Patterning. Barrett (1990) defines deliberative mutual patterning as, "The continuous process whereby the nurse with the client patterns the environmental field to promote harmony related to health events. In the deliberative mutual patterning phase of the Rogerian practice methodology, the nurse facilitates the client's actualization of potentials for health and well-being" (pp. 33–34). The nurse and client take deliberate actions to direct the actions, behaviors, thoughts, and inevitable changes that occur.

After pattern appraisal, the nurse and client participate in a deliberate mutual patterning process which facilitates knowing participation in change. The teaching heuristic used in the Personalized Nursing practice model designed to be used to facilitate deliberative mutual pattern change is the Personalized Nursing LIGHT Model. The acronym LIGHT is used twice: First, to remind nurses and caregivers of their roles in developing pattern changes, and second, as an acronym for a process clients can be taught to improve well-being (see Table 13.3).

Facets of the LIGHT Model Process for Deliberative Mutual Patterning

• Bonding	Love the client. Intend to be helpful. Give your care gently.
• Assess Well-Being	Help the client identify barriers to and improve his/her well-being.
• Teach the LIGHT Model	Teach a healing process and help clients plan the first step to deliberate pattern change.

Awareness Transformation

Nurses who deliberately focus on their value for their clients (e.g., L-Love the client) facilitate a mutual awareness of the clients' value and talents. Clients often feel alone and isolated with their pain. They don't feel they are people of value. By focusing on a client's value, nurses using the LIGHT Model facilitate an increased awareness within the client of their

Table 13.3   Personalized Nursing LIGHT Model

Nurses and Caregivers	You
Love the client.	Love yourself.
Intend to help.	Identify a concern.
Give Care Gently.	Give yourself a goal.
Help the client improve well-being.	Have confidence and help yourself.
Teach the process.	Take positive action.

own sense of value and of the mutual processing of their human energy field with their infinite environmental energy field. Malinski (1993) states that integrality is ever present (p. 57). She says that one can focus awareness on integrality which, although ever present, is not always fully experienced. She says Therapeutic Touch, for example, is a way to focus awareness integrality between the client and his or her environmental field.

We postulate that nurses and clients use the Personalized Nursing LIGHT Model to focus their attention on the client's value, unique talents, and on the integrality of the client and the universe. Drug-addicted individuals do not experience an awareness of integrality unless they are "high" (e.g., in a higher frequency alternative reality).

A client's increased awareness of his or her mutual process with the infinite universe of energy is likely to be associated with an increased sense of well-being. The pattern manifestations associated with an improved sense of well-being that emerge from this mutual process reflect heightened awareness, higher frequency energy patterns, and more diverse energy fields. With this new higher frequency awareness (illumination), clients can "see" many options and possible actions formerly "invisible" to them. This awareness allows clients to examine honestly their lifestyle in relation to their drug use and experience of pain that to them appears, at times, to consume their very being. This insight can be an awakening to the healing powers within themselves enabling them to recognize alternative options available and to participate knowingly in making choices that accelerate change and promote well-being.

SUMMARY

Clients who received nursing care with the LIGHT Model improved their well-being, which was associated with a decrease in high-risk drug injecting behaviors. Standard care clients who did not receive LIGHT Model care only knew one way to improve well-being—injecting more drugs. There was no positive association between improved well-being and a decrease in high-risk behaviors in the group of clients who received *only* standard care treatment. By helping clients improve well-being, nurses assisted them to see more options and possibilities.

Nurses practicing the Personalized Nursing LIGHT Model deliberately bring an awareness—a perceived openness—to the environmental field of the client with which they are integral. The nurse and client participate in purposive patterning of the human/environmental field. Within the presence of the nurse's openness and awareness of the client's value, the client becomes more open and aware of their individual value and their ongoing connection with a universe of energy integral with himself or herself. With a comprehension of this ever-present, dynamic mutual process of human/environmental fields, a client's awareness of options in life increases. More behavior choices appear as possible.

Malinski (1993, p. 52) suggests ". . . higher frequency knowing participation may be part of the acceleration in change theorized by Rogers." She goes on to say "diversity accelerates with higher frequency phenomena . . ." She concludes that "while specific outcomes can't be predicted by nursing-based health patterning modalities, this may be the basis for the assertion that the experience is likely to be beneficial to the client." Our data show that having an experience with the Personalized Nursing LIGHT practice model of nursing is beneficial to clients.

REFERENCES

Andersen, M. D. (1986). Personalized nursing: An intervention model for use with drug dependent women in an emergency room. *International Journal of Addictions, 21*(1), 105-122.

Andersen, M. D., & Braunstein, M. S. (1992). Conceptions of therapy: Personalized nursing LIGHT model with chemically dependent female offenders. In T. Mieczkowski (Ed.), *Drugs, crime, and social policy: Research, issues, and concerns* (pp. 250-262). Needham Heights, MA: Allyn & Bacon.

Andersen, M. D., & Smereck, G. A. D. (1989). Personalized nursing LIGHT model. *Nursing Science Quarterly, 2* 120-130.

Andersen, M. D., & Smereck, G. A. D. (1992). The consciousness rainbow: An explication of Rogerian field pattern manifestations. *Nursing Science Quarterly, 5* 72-79.

Andersen, M. D., & Smereck, G. A. D. (1994). Personalized nursing: A science-based model of the art of nursing. In M. Madrid & E. Barrett (Eds.), *Rogers' scientific art of nursing practice* (pp. 261-283). New York: NLN Press.

Andersen, M. D., Smereck, G. A. D., & Braunstein, M. S. (1993). LIGHT model: An effective intervention model to change high-risk AIDS behaviors among hard-to-reach urban drug users. *America Journal of Drug and Alcohol Abuse, 19*(3), 309-325.

Andersen, M. D., Smereck, G. A. D., & Hockman, E. M. (1996). Effect of a nursing outreach intervention to drug users in Detroit, Michigan. *Journal of Drug Issues, 26*(3), 619-634.

Andrews, F. M., & Withey, S. B. (1976). *Social indicators of well-being.* New York: Plenum.

Aristotle. (1984). Nicomachean ethics: Physics: Eudemian ethics. In J. Barnes (Ed.), *The complete works of Aristotle.* Princeton, NJ: Princeton University Press.

Barrett, E. A. M. (1988). Using Rogers' science of unitary human beings in nursing practice. *Nursing Science Quarterly, 1,* 50–51.

Barrett, E. A. M. (1990). Rogers' science-based nursing practice. In E. A. M. Barrett (Ed.), *Visions of Rogers' science-based nursing* (pp. 31–44). New York: NLN Press.

Braunstein, M. S. (1993). Sampling a hidden population: Noninstitutionalized drug users. *AIDS Education & Prevention, 5*(2), 131–140.

Coyle, S. L. (1993). *The NIDA HIV counseling and education intervention model: Intervention manual* (NIH Pub. No. 93-3508). Rockville, MD: U.S. Department of Health and Human Services.

Dowling-Guyer, S., Johnson, M. E., Fisher, D. G., Andersen, M., Watters, J., Williams, M., Kotranski, L., Booth, R., Rhodes, F., Weatherby, N., Estrada, A. L., Fleming, D., Deren, S., & Tortu, S. (1994). Reliability of drug users' self-reported HIV risk behaviors and validity of self-reported recent drug use. *Assessment, 4,* 383–392.

Hockman, E. M. (1994). *The construct of meaning through data reduction, aggregation, and refinement.* Paper presented at the Second Science Symposium, Flagstaff, AZ.

Malinski, V. M. (1993). Therapeutic touch: The view from Rogerian nursing science. *Visions: The Journal of Rogerian Nursing Science. 1,* 45–54.

McLellan, A. T., Luborsky, L., Cacciola, T., Griffith, J., McGahen, P., & Obriun, C. P. (1985). Guide to the Addiction Severity Index: Backgound administration and field testing results (DHHS Publication No. ADM85-1419). Rockville, MD: National Institute on Drug Abuse.

Needle, R., Weatherby, N., Chitwood, D., Booth, R., Watters, J., Fisher, D. G., Brown, B., Cesari, H., Williams, M. L., Andersen, M., & Braunstein, M. (1995). Reliability of self-reported HIV risk behaviors of drug users. *Psychology of Addictive Behaviors, 9*(4), 242–250.

Personalized Nursing Corporation. (1995, September). *Final report* (National Institute on Drug Abuse Grant No. 5 U01 DA06903). Detroit, MI: M. D. Andersen & G. A. D. Smereck.

Rogers, M. E. (1986). Science of unitary human beings. In V. Malinski (Ed.), *Explorations on Martha Rogers' science of unitary human beings.* Norwalk, CT: Appleton-Century-Croft.

Rogers, M. E. (1990). Nursing: Science of unitary irreducible, human beings: Update 1990. In E. A. M. Barrett (Ed.), *Visions of Rogers' science-based nursing*(pp. 5–11). New York: NLN Press.

Weatherby, N. L., Needle, R., Cesari, H., Booth, R., McCoy, C. B., Watters, J. K., Williams, M., & Chitwood, D. D. (1994). Validity of self-reported drug use among injection drug users and crack cocaine users recruited through street outreach. *Evaluation and Program Planning, 17*(4), 347–355.

14

Using Rogers' Model to Study Sleep-Wake Pattern Changes in Older Women

Juanita Watson

*T*he sleep-wake patterns of older adults have been found by numerous non-Rogerian researchers to be different from those of younger adults. Sleep at night is lighter and more fragmented. Older adults tend to wake up more frequently at night; some take more daytime naps. Time spent sleeping per day varies. The onset of sleep pattern changes usually occurs when people are in their 50s (Webb, 1989). In this chapter, a study is presented in which Rogers' (1970, 1992) model was used as the framework for explaining these changes.

THEORETICAL BACKGROUND

Non-Rogerian researchers have proposed two principal theories to explain the sleep-wake pattern changes in older adults. Most commonly, the disrupted sleep-wake rhythms are viewed as evidence of the biologic deterioration associated with aging. Neurological alterations that lead to destabilization of biological rhythms, along with various physical problems, are included as causes of sleep pattern changes according to this theoretical perspective (Colling, 1983; Kedas, Lux, & Amodeo, 1989). Others think that, in addition to biological deterioration, sleep pattern changes in older adults occur as a result of changes in job, family, and social pressures, as well as from worry, anxiety, and depression (Prinz, Vitiello, Raskind, & Thorpy, 1990; Webb, 1989). Neither of these approaches, however, fully explains these commonly observed sleep pattern changes.

Rogers (1970, 1992) has offered a different way to look at changes in sleep-wake rhythms. According to the conceptual model, sleep-wake rhythm is a manifestation of human field patterning. These manifestations, not chronological age, are used to describe the change process in unitary human beings and include: longer sleeping to longer waking to beyond waking; slower motion to faster motion to seemingly continuous motion; and time experienced as slower to time experienced as faster to a sense of timelessness (Rogers, 1992). Change is continuous from conception through dying and is characterized by increasing diversity and innovation of the human field pattern.

As human fields evolve, sleep-wake patterns become increasingly diverse and waking periods lengthen (Rogers, 1992). Such changes may occur in individuals of all ages and are not limited to the elderly (Rogers, 1980); however, when these changes are observed in older adults they would be viewed as "normal" variations, not evidence of physical or psychological problems. Further, not all individuals manifest the same variation in sleep-wake rhythms. As Rogers (1992) notes, "the more diverse field patterns evolve more rapidly than the less diverse ones . . . [and] individual differences multiply" (p. 32). Indeed, a high degree of variability in sleep-wake rhythms among individuals has been noted by non-Rogerian sleep theorists and researchers (Hayter, 1983; Moorcroft, 1989; Webb, 1989). In the current investigation, variability in sleep-wake rhythms was proposed as an indicator of changing diversity of the human sleep-wake experience, with a greater number of sleep-wake events indicating a higher degree of diversity, as measured with a modified Sleep Chart (Lewis & Masterson, 1957; Tune, 1969a, 1969b).

Change in the human sleep-wake manifestation of patterning is conceptualized as encompassing experiences beyond sleeping and waking (i.e., "beyond waking" experiences). Although "beyond waking" is not defined by Rogers, she cites paranormal and meditative experiences as examples (Rogers, 1992). Human sleep-wake rhythms cannot be fully explored without consideration of beyond waking manifestations.

In the current investigation, dreaming was said to be a beyond waking experience. As Rogers (1970) has stated, "Dreams are often noted to be associated with paranormal phenomena . . . [and] provide a further means whereby integration and patterning of life occur" (p. 72). Dreaming has also been described by others (Dement, 1976; Hartocollis, 1980; Namilov, 1982) as being similar to or having characteristics of those experiences considered to be beyond waking manifestations in Rogers' model. Chuman (1983) and Hobson and McCarley (1977) have suggested that the human sleep-wake rhythm be viewed in relation to three principal states: waking, sleeping, and dreaming. Sleeping and dreaming are not, however, mutually exclusive experiences. Dreaming may occur during all stages of sleep. As the human field evolves, its pattern becomes increasingly diverse. Thus, the degree of diversity in dream experience was proposed as an indicator of field pattern change in beyond waking manifestations. The Assessment of Dream Experience (Watson, 1993), was developed to measure this variable.

Each of the manifestations of patterning in unitary human beings represents an indicator of the human field in its entirety (Rogers, 1992). These pattern characteristics are postulated "to evolve consonantly with one another in unitary human development" (Cowling, 1983, p. 2). That is, "as change occurs in one part of the [human] field, change takes place in the whole field" (Phillips, 1989, p. 58) and is similarly evidenced in each of the manifestations. In this study, diversity of sleep-wake rhythm and diversity of dream experience were compared with human field motion and time experience, two manifestations of patterning that have been validated in previous Rogerian studies (Butcher & Parker, 1988; Ference, 1979; Ludomirski, 1984; Macrae, 1982). These latter two variables were measured with the Human Field Motion Tool (Ference, 1979) and the Time Metaphor Test (Knapp & Garbutt, 1958), respectively.

PURPOSES, PROBLEM, AND HYPOTHESIS

The main purpose of conducting the study was to explore a new approach to explaining sleep-wake pattern changes in older adults, and more specifically, to verify Rogers' ideas. An additional purpose was to investigate whether diversity of sleep-wake rhythm and dream experience are indicators of change in the human field pattern by exploring their relationships with human field motion and time experience. The research problem was: What are the relationships of sleep-wake rhythm and dream experience to human field motion and time experience?

The hypothesis was that there would be at least one significant relationship between the set of scores of sleep-wake rhythm and dream experience and the set of scores of human field motion and time experience. The criteria variables, sleep-wake rhythm and dream experience, were handled as a set because they were postulated to represent the longer sleeping/longer waking/beyond waking manifestation of patterning.

METHOD

Sample

In this descriptive study, the convenience sample consisted of 66 women, ages 60 to 83 ($M = 71.2$). Chronological age was used to delimit the sample, so that the results of the study could be compared with those from non-Rogerian studies. The study was limited to women to control for reported gender differences in objective and subjective measures of sleep-wake rhythms (Rediehs, Reis, & Creason, 1990). No participant was confined to any type of health or custodial care facility with enforced, institutionally defined routines. Volunteers were sought from various groups and organizations in the community. Numerous factors such as drugs and alcohol, worry and anxiety, and various presleep activities are known to affect sleep-wake patterns. Although the sample was not delimited in relation to these factors, data were obtained and analyzed for possible effects on the main variables. The sample size was sufficient to detect a medium effect ($f^2 = .15$) with a power greater than .80 in multiple regression analysis at the .05 level of significance (Cohen, 1977).

Most participants (86.4%) were educated beyond the high school level; 40.9 percent held at least a Master's degree, and 84.9 percent reported taking long walks on a regular basis. The majority of the sample (68.2%) rated their health as good to excellent, and 70.4 percent reported that 10 or more days of the 14-day study had been typical for them (i.e., they went about their usual activities with the usual demands on their personal schedules).

Instruments

The instruments used included: (1) a demographic questionnaire, (2) a modified Sleep Chart that the participants maintained for 14 days, (3) the Assessment of Dream Experience, (4) the Human Field Motion Tool, and (5) the Time Metaphor Test. Validity and reliability of the instruments were ascertained prior to implementation of the study (Watson, 1993).

Procedure

Participants gave written consent, completed the demographic question-naire, and began maintaining the Sleep Chart. They were instructed to com-plete the remaining instruments after the Sleep Chart had been kept for two weeks. The Assessment of Dream Experience had to be completed after the Sleep Chart, since the directions for use indicated that the participants should rate what their dreams had been like over the preceding two weeks. For participant convenience, the Human Field Motion Tool and the Time Metaphor Test were completed after the Sleep Chart had been maintained.

RESULTS

Sleep-Wake Pattern Characteristics of the Sample

The majority of the sample (75.8%) reported that they slept six to eight hours per day; 13.6 percent slept less than six and 9.1 percent slept more than eight. The majority of participants (72.7%) did not share a bed or bedroom, and 66.7 percent did not consider themselves to be under stress that interfered with their sleep. Neither alcohol nor tobacco was used on a regular basis by 86.4 percent of the sample.

The most frequent responses to the question, Do you do anything spe-cial to get to sleep?, were reading (63.3%), praying (56.1%), watching tele-vision/videotapes (42.4%), or listening to radio/records/tapes (24.2%). Only three participants (4.6%) took sleeping pills, while nine (13.6%) took other medications such as sedatives, antidepressants, aspirin, and antacids. Five respondents (7.6%) took a pain reliever to get to sleep. Overall, 25.8 percent took medications to get to sleep.

The majority of the sample (72.7%) indicated awakening at night "al-most always" or "frequently." Half of the participants (51.5%) indicated that they rarely or never took naps, however, 21.2 percent reported at least one or more daily naps. Forty-three participants (65.2%) indicated that their sleep patterns had changed since middle adulthood. The type of sleep pattern change indicated by most participants (55.8%) was more frequent awakenings at night, and the age at which these sleep pattern changes occurred in 39.5 percent of the participants was 60 to 69 years. These sleep pattern characteristics are similar to those reported by other sleep researchers (Bonnett & Rosa, 1987; Dement, Miles, & Carskadon, 1982; Hayter, 1983; Kronholm & Hyyppa, 1985; Minors, Rabbitt, Worht-ington, & Waterhouse, 1989; Shaver & Giblin, 1989; Snyder-Halpern & Verran, 1987; Stone, 1989; Webb, 1989).

Rogers' (1992) statement that "sleep-wake frequencies become more varied" (p. 32) is supported by the finding of increased nocturnal awakenings. Her contention that "the aged sleep less" (Rogers, 1986, p. 7), is not supported by these findings, and as Stone (1989) notes, "the issue of whether total sleep time changes in [older adults] is not yet clear" (p. 367).

An unexpected finding was the degree of satisfaction with sleep patterns, especially in light of the reported frequency of nocturnal awakenings and changes in sleep-wake patterns since middle age. The majority of participants (71.2%) indicated that they were "very" to "moderately" satisfied with their current sleep patterns. Other sleep researchers have reported that older individuals have more subjective complaints about their sleep patterns than younger adults (Dement et al., 1982; Webb, 1989). Moreover, women have been reported to have more subjective complaints than men (Kronholm & Hyyppa, 1985; Rediehs et al., 1990). Webb (1989) notes, however, that "there is increasing evidence that older persons, in the face of these [sleep pattern changes] do not report untoward consequences, view them with alarm, or seek treatment in relation to them" (p. 285). Snyder-Halpern and Verran (1987), for example, found that "older subjects reported higher sleep quality and a feeling of being rested" (p. 161), despite significant increases in mid-sleep awakenings. Further, Webb (1989) states that subjective reports of sleep disturbances may simply "affirm the awareness of old persons to the objective changes in sleep" (p. 282), and may not necessarily indicate either pathology or dissatisfaction. The results of the current investigation support these findings and interpretations, and provide some empirical support for Rogers' (1986, 1992) position that sleep-wake pattern changes are normal phenomena.

Main Variables

The distributions of scores for the four main variables were approximately normal, without excessive skewness or kurtosis. This suggests that the higher than normal levels of education and physical activity did not influence the results with respect to the hypothesis.

A significant positive correlation ($r = .2945$, $p < .05$) was found between the two dependent variables, sleep-wake rhythm and dream experience. There were no significant correlations of these variables with either of the independent variables, human field motion and time experience, nor were the independent variables correlated with each other. Because of the lack of correlation between the independent and dependent variables, regression and canonical correlation analyses were not significant (Munro, Visintainer, & Page, 1986). The hypothesis was not supported.

The positive correlation between sleep-wake rhythm and dream experience is promising in terms of finding a way to measure Rogers' construct of the longer sleeping/longer waking/beyond waking manifestation of patterning. The fact that the shared variance was only 8.75 percent suggests the need for further investigation of additional variables which may be indicants of this manifestation of patterning, especially beyond waking manifestations. This researcher offers a definition of beyond waking experiences: Complex human field phenomena that occur during periods of both waking and sleeping, yet transcend both, and involve the perception of pandimensional realities in "an infinite domain without limit" (Rogers, 1992, p. 31). Examples of beyond waking experiences, in addition to meditation and paranormal phenomena already identified by Rogers (1992) are: dreaming, lucid dreaming, daydreaming, guided imagery, out-of-body and near-death experiences, and spirituality. Qualitative and quantitative studies should be conducted to further explore the nature and meaning of beyond waking experiences within the context of the Rogerian model. Perhaps an instrument could be developed that incorporates the variety of experiences that are linked to the beyond waking construct.

The lack of relationship between human field motion and time experience was probably due to problems with the instruments, and not due to a lack of theoretical relationship between the two. The fact that there were no relationships between either of these two variables with either of the dependent variables, sleep-wake rhythm and dream experience, also may be the result of measurement problems, especially with respect to time experience and human field motion.

Problems with scoring and interpretation of scores on the Time Metaphor Test have been addressed elsewhere (Watson, 1996). Problems with the Human Field Motion Tool, in general, were: (1) lack of understanding of the instrument by the participants, especially with respect to terminology, concepts to be rated, and use of the semantic differential format; (2) questions about the instrument's factorial validity; and (3) issues pertaining to how scores on the instrument are determined. An additional problem is the relevance of the concepts rated to Rogers' (1992) current version of her model. For example, one of the concepts rated is, "my field expansion." This concept is derived from Rogers' (1970) early ideas that human energy fields had boundaries and that these boundaries fluctuated. Rogers (1992) now posits that energy fields are infinite and boundaryless. Thus, of the two concepts rated on the instrument, one is no longer valid theoretically within the conceptual model for which it was designed to be used.

Supplementary Findings

Supplementary analysis revealed a small but statistically significant positive correlation ($r = .2863$, $p = .05$) between age and time experience. This was not as theoretically expected and may have been due to characteristics of the sample such as perceived good health, satisfaction with sleep patterns, ability to provide own personal care, and involvement in clubs, organizations, and religious activities. There were no correlations between age and the other main variables.

NURSING IMPLICATIONS

Nursing implications of the study have to do with gaining a better understanding of normal sleep pattern variations and communicating this information to nurses and consumers of nursing services in a variety of settings. Nurses working in hospitals and extended care facilities need to understand that it may not be reasonable to expect clients to sleep throughout the night. Nursing modalities for clients who are awake and practices to promote sleep at night should be re-examined, particularly from Rogers' (1992) theoretical perspective. Staffing patterns at night may need to be changed. Nurses may also use the information from this study to teach clients about sleep pattern changes that typically occur in middle-aged and older adults. Such information may help to alleviate some of the frustration experienced when unable to sleep like a young adult and it may help to avoid dependence on pharmacologic sleep inducers. Further, knowing about sleep pattern changes may be helpful to family members in multigenerational households.

RECOMMENDATIONS FOR FURTHER RESEARCH

Additional investigations of the longer sleeping/longer waking/beyond waking manifestation of patterning should be conducted to further clarify and verify Rogers' (1992) theoretical approach to explaining variations in sleep-wake rhythms, as well as to further explore the nature and meaning of beyond waking experiences. There is also a need for validation of existing instruments and clarification of theoretical and measurement issues pertaining to their use. Development of new instruments that address the longer sleeping/longer waking/beyond waking manifestation of patterning should be considered.

REFERENCES

Bonnett, M. H., & Rosa, R. R. (1987). Sleep and performance in young adults and older normals and insomniacs during acute sleep loss and recovery. *Biological Psychology, 25,* 153–172.

Butcher, H. K., & Parker, N. I. (1988). Guided imagery within Rogers' science of unitary human beings: An experimental study. *Nursing Science Quarterly, 1,* 103–110.

Chuman, M. A. (1983). The neurological basis of sleep. *Heart & Lung, 12,* 177–182.

Cohen, J. (1977). *Statistical power analysis.* New York: Academic Press.

Colling, J. (1983). Sleep disturbances in aging: A theoretic and empirical analysis. *Advances in Nursing Science, 6*(1), 36–44.

Cowling. W. R. (1983). *The relationship of mystical experience, differentiation, and creativity in college students.* Unpublished doctoral dissertation, New York University, New York.

Dement, W. C. (1976). *Some must watch while some must sleep.* San Francisco, CA: San Francisco Book.

Dement, W. C., Miles, L. E., & Carskadon, M. A. (1982). "White paper" on sleep in aging. *Journal of the American Geriatrics Society, 30,* 25–50.

Ference, H. M. (1979). *The relationship of time experience, creativity traits, differentiation, and human field motion.* Unpublished doctoral dissertation, New York University, New York.

Hartocollis, P. (1980). Time and the dream. *Journal of the American Psychoanalytic Association, 28,* 861–867.

Hayter, J. (1983). Sleep behaviors of older persons. *Nursing Research, 32,* 242–246.

Hobson, J. A., & McCarley, R. W. (1977). The brain as dream state generator: An activation-synthesis hypothesis of the dream process. *American Journal of Psychiatry, 134,* 1335–1348.

Kedas, A., Lux, W., & Amodeo, S. (1989). A critical review of aging and sleep research. *Western Journal of Nursing Research, 11,* 196–206.

Kronholm, E., & Hyyppa, M. T. (1985). Age-related sleep habits and retirement. *Annals of Clinical Research, 17,* 257–264.

Knapp, R. H., & Garbutt, J. T. (1958). Time imagery and the achievement motive. *Journal of Personality, 26,* 426–434.

Lewis, H. E., & Masterson, J. P. (1957). Sleep and wakefulness in the Arctic. *Lancet, 272,* 1262–1266.

Ludomirski, B. G. (1984). *The relationship between environmental energy wave frequency pattern manifest in red light and blue light and human field motion in adult individuals with visual sensory perception and those with total blindness.* Unpublished doctoral dissertation, New York University, New York.

Macrae, J. (1982). *A comparison between meditating subjects and non-meditating subjects on time experience and human field motion.* Unpublished doctoral dissertation, New York, New York.

Minors, D. S., Rabbitt, P. A., Worthington, H., & Waterhouse, J. M. (1989). Variation in meals and sleep-wake activity patterns in aged subjects: Its relevance to circadian rhythm studies. *Chronobiology International, 6,* 139-148.

Moorcroft, W. H. (1989). *Sleep, dreaming, and sleep disorders: An introduction.* Lanham, MD: University Press of America.

Munro, B. H., Visintainer, M. A., & Page, E. B. (1986). *Statistical methods for health care research.* Philadelphia: Lippincott.

Namilov, V. V. (1982). *Realms of the unconscious: The enchanted frontier.* Philadelphia: ISF Press.

Phillips, J. R. (1989). Science of unitary human beings: Changing research perspectives. *Nursing Science Quarterly, 2,* 57-59.

Prinz, P. N., Vitiello, M. V., Raskind, M. A., & Thorpy, M. J. (1990). Geriatrics: Sleep disorders and aging. *New England Journal of Medicine, 323,* 520-526.

Rediehs, M. H., Reis, J. S., & Creason, N. S. (1990). Sleep in old age: Focus on gender differences. *Sleep, 13,* 410-424.

Rogers, M. E. (1970). *An introduction to the theoretical basis of nursing.* Philadelphia: F.A. Davis.

Rogers, M. E. (1980). Nursing: A science of unitary man. In J. Riehl & Sr. C. Roy (Eds.), *Conceptual models for nursing practice* (2nd ed. pp. 329-337). Norwalk, CT: Appleton-Century-Crofts.

Rogers, M. E., (1986). Science of unitary human beings. In V. M. Malinski (Ed.), *Explorations on Martha Rogers' science of unitary human beings* (pp. 3-8). Norwalk, CT: Appleton-Century-Crofts.

Rogers, M. E. (1992). Nursing science and the space age. *Nursing Science Quarterly, 5*(1), 27-34.

Shaver, J. L., & Giblin, E. G (1989). Sleep. *Annual Review of Nursing Research, 7,* 71-93.

Snyder-Halpern, R., & Verran, J. A. (1987). Instrumentation to describe subjective sleep characteristics in healthy subjects. *Research in Nursing & Health, 10,* 155-163.

Stone, W. S. (1989). Sleep and aging in animals. *Clinics in Geriatric Medicine, 5,* 363-379.

Tune, G. S. (1969a). Sleep and wakefulness in 509 normal human adults. *British Journal of Medical Psychology, 42,* 75-80.

Tune, G. S. (1969b). The influence of age and temperament on the adult human sleep-wakefulness pattern. *British Journal of Psychology, 60,* 431-441.

Watson, J. (1993). *The relationships of sleep-wake rhythm, dream experience, human field motion, and time experience in older women.* Unpublished doctoral dissertation, New York University, New York. (University Microfilms No. 94-11208).

Watson, J. (1996). Issues with measuring time experience in Rogers' conceptual model. *Visions: Journal of Rogerian Nursing Science, 4*(1), 31-40.

Webb, W. B. (1989). Age-related changes in sleep. *Clinics in Geriatric Medicine, 5,* 275-287.

15

Power, Perceived Health, and Life Satisfaction in Adults with Long-Term Care Needs

Martha A. McNiff

*D*isability interferes with the lives of over 35 million Americans and is considered the country's foremost public health concern (Pope & Tarlov, 1991). Proponents of the medical model treat the dysfunctional parts of the disabled using a reductionist, causal approach to human beings and their environment. Martha E. Rogers (1970, 1992) provided an alternative conceptual model. She encouraged healthcare professionals to view people with long-term care needs not as those with "broken parts" but rather as unitary human energy fields who are different from the sum of their parts and integral with the environmental energy field. From the perspective of Rogers' model, disability can be viewed as a transformation in the continuous mutual process of the human and environmental energy field pattern.

According to Rogers (1992), pattern—the distinguishing characteristic of human energy fields—changes continuously and is an abstraction known by its manifestations. Power, perceived health, and life satisfaction are pattern manifestations that emerge from the increasingly diverse continuous mutual human-environmental energy field process. This researcher explored the relationships of and differences in these manifestations in people with and those without long-term care needs. Adults with long-term care needs were defined as people institutionalized in a physical rehabilitation long-term care facility, unable to perform one or more essential activities of daily living (ADL), and who required assistance with activities necessary to maintain independence (Friedland, 1990). Adults without long-term care needs were employees in the same facility, and were able to perform ADL and activities necessary to maintain independence.

POWER

Power is generally defined in causal terms as a coercive force (Olsen, 1970), an authority legitimized by law or social norms (Weber, 1970), or as a resource (Marx, 1970). Social learning theorists portray power as control, and note that people who believe they control their own destiny strive to improve their environment (Rotter, 1982). Barrett (1983) derived a theory of power from the Science of Unitary Human Beings, conceptualizing power as a manifestation of change. In the theory of accelerating change, Rogers (1986) states that field patterns become increasingly diverse. According to Ference (1979), human field motion (HFM), a concept based on Rogers' science, represents increasingly diverse change. Barrett (1983), who found a relationship between power and HFM, believed that power reflected the nature of change, and concluded that as the life process proceeds, so does the capacity to participate knowingly in change. Power is "the capacity to participate knowingly in the nature of change characterizing the continuous patterning of the human and environmental fields" (Barrett, 1990, p. 108). Human field pattern characteristics of power are awareness of self and environment, choosing alternatives, acting intentionally, and involvement in creating change (Barrett, 1983).

Feelings associated with HFM imply characteristics of health. The relationship between power and HFM suggests a relationship between power and health. Ference (1986) states that higher frequency or increased HFM is characterized by feeling unresponsive to physical environmental events, feeling exuberant, relaxed, revitalized, strong, bright, and active. These feelings are similar to reports of health. Lower frequency or decreased HFM is characterized by feeling weak, dragging, sleepy, dull, and passive (Ference, 1986, pp. 101–102). Such feelings are often evident in illness. People who have a positive perception of their health tend to participate in health-promoting behaviors (Jones, 1991). Health-promoting behavior indicates involvement in creating change in one's life, a characteristic of power, and this behavior suggests a relationship between power and health.

HEALTH

Health is a universal phenomenon which varies within and among individuals throughout life (Hurrelmann, 1989). Advocates of the biomedical model define health as the absence of disease (Sobel, 1979). In the sociological model, health is the ability to perform roles and tasks expected by society (Parsons, 1979). Supporters of the systems model view health as the ability to adapt to environmental challenges (Brody & Sobel, 1979). Rogers (1970) refers to health and illness as manifestations of the life process. According to Rogers (1990), "unitary human health signifies an irreducible human field manifestation . . . [which] cannot be measured by the parameters of biology or physics or the social sciences and the like" (p. 10). Human field behavior of power indicating change is evident in health. Health is characterized by awareness (Fitzpatrick, 1983), choice (Madrid & Winstead-Fry, 1986), and participation in life (Siegel, 1986). In Rogers' model, health can be defined as a human field pattern manifestation, emerging from the increasingly diverse human/environmental energy field process, characterized by changing patterns that a person describes as best or worst health. Perceived health is a person's self-report of current health and it includes various characteristics.

LIFE SATISFACTION

Life satisfaction is unique to each person (Conte & Salamon, 1982) and is considered the most crucial indicator of quality of life and well-being (George & Bearon, 1980). Studies of life satisfaction are often based on reductionist models whose proponents attribute life satisfaction to such factors as income (Spreitzer & Snyder, 1974), social support (Levitt, Clark, Rotton, & Finley, 1987), and religious practices (Hunsberger, 1985). Campbell, Converse, and Rodgers (1976) believe that experience and behavior emerge from the person-environment interaction, and that individuals subjectively define their life satisfaction. They define life satisfaction as "the generalized sense of well-being with life as currently experienced" (Campbell et al., 1976, p. 50). This perspective is congruent with Rogers' view of the integrality of human beings and their environment.

Life satisfaction is a human field pattern manifestation emerging from the increasingly diverse continuous mutual process of the human and environmental energy fields. Satisfaction is characterized as perceiving life as enjoyable, full, rewarding, bringing out one's best, interesting, hopeful, friendly, and worthwhile. Dissatisfaction is characterized as perceiving life as miserable, empty, disappointing, not giving one much chance, boring, discouraging, lonely, and useless (Campbell et al., 1976).

Researchers have linked life satisfaction to power and health. Rizzo (1990) reported a positive correlation between Barrett's Power as Knowing Participation in Change Tool—a measure of change—and life satisfaction in elderly adults. Rizzo concluded that as people participate in the patterning of the human-environmental field process through their choices, and experience their participation and choices positively, they manifest a pattern of life satisfaction. Reed (1987) confirmed positive relationships between life satisfaction and self-rated health in terminally ill hospitalized cancer patients, nonterminally ill hospitalized patients, and healthy nonhospitalized patients. Reed observed that even the dying have a potential for well-being.

HYPOTHESES AND RESEARCH QUESTIONS

Hypotheses stated that power, perceived health, and life satisfaction would be positively related in both adults with long-term care needs and in adults without long-term care needs. Since this is a new realm of study within Rogers' Science of Unitary Human Beings, research questions were asked in order to examine differences between the two groups in power, perceived health, and life satisfaction, and to determine if these relationships varied as a function of long-term care need (McNiff, 1996).

METHOD

This descriptive study was conducted in a municipal physical rehabilitation long-term care facility. A convenience sample of adults with long-term care needs ($N = 68$) was obtained from among facility residents. A second convenience sample of adults without long-term care needs ($N = 68$) was obtained from among employees within the same facility.

Participants were adults, at least 18 years of age, who understood and could communicate in English, and had a minimum of a high school education. To allow for acclimation to the environment, people admitted to or employed by the facility for less than one month were excluded from the study. Since changes in pattern manifestations were explored from the perspective of adults with acquired long-term care needs, people with congenital or developmental disabilities were excluded from the study. People who met the criteria and gave informed consent responded to background questions and the Power as Knowing Participation in Change Tool (Barrett, 1983), the Cantril (1965) ladder for health, and the Index of Well-Being (Campbell et al., 1976) for life satisfaction.

The majority of participants with long-term care needs were unmarried black males, mean age 46, with vocational or high school educations. The majority of these participants (64.7%) sustained spinal cord injuries (38.2%) or cerebral vascular accidents (26.5%). Others evidenced a variety of health problems, such as amputations due to diabetes (13.2%), chronic obstructive pulmonary disease (7.4%), and multiple sclerosis (5.9%). The remaining 8.8 percent of people with long-term care needs had diverse conditions, such as bone cancer, hip fractures, and Pott's disease. The majority of participants without long-term care needs were married white females, mean age 41, with an associate or higher college degree.

FINDINGS

Pearson product-moment correlations were used to test the hypotheses. A one-tailed t-test determined the statistical significance of the correlations. The first hypothesis stated that power, perceived health, and life satisfaction would be positively related in adults with long-term care needs. The relationships between power and life satisfaction ($r = .60$) and between life satisfaction and perceived health ($r = .41$) were statistically significant ($p < .001$). The relationship of power and perceived health ($r = .24$) was not statistically significant. The first hypothesis was partially supported.

The second hypothesis stated that power, perceived health, and life satisfaction would be positively related in adults without long-term care needs. The relationships between power and perceived health ($r = .42$), perceived health and life satisfaction ($r = .52$), and power and life satisfaction ($r = .63$) were statistically significant ($p = .001$).

Research questions asked if there were differences in power, perceived health, and life satisfaction between adults with and those without long-term care needs, and if the relationships among these manifestations varied as a function of long-term care need. Research questions were analyzed using an analysis of covariance to control for differences found between the groups in age, annual income, employment status, ethnicity, frequency of prayer or meditation, and gender. No differences were found between adults with and adults without long-term care needs in power ($F = .006$, $df = 1$, 128, $p = .940$), perceived health ($F = .025$, $df = 1$, 128, $p = .874$), or life satisfaction ($F = .335$, $df = 1$, 128, $p = .563$). No statistically significant differences were found between the two groups in the relationships of the main variables.

DISCUSSION

This researcher supports Rogers' belief in the unitary nature of human beings. Amid various health patterns, people with long-term care needs participated knowingly in change and manifested well-being in their lives. Manifestations of well-being may indicate increasingly diverse field patterning in people who are able to transcend disability through a pandimensional reality. People without long-term care needs manifested power and concomitant changes in their pattern manifestations of health and life satisfaction. The two groups did not differ significantly in power, perceived health, or life satisfaction, or in the relationships of these variables. This incredible finding further demonstrates the unitary nature of the human energy field.

Positive correlations between perceived health and life satisfaction may indicate that these concepts are complementary dimensions of well-being. This assumption is further supported by an overlap in responses to open-ended questions on the background information form that asked participants to define health and life satisfaction. Participants described health in physical and psychological terms, as independence in ADL, engaging in health practices, having a positive value, and including a spiritual dimension. Descriptions of health by people with long-term care needs often reflected their unique needs. A ventilator-dependent participant responded poignantly that "health is breathing and having nothing wrong with your body." A stroke victim defined health as "walking right, talking right, eating, sleeping, (and) having all your senses working."

Descriptions of life satisfaction included fulfilling interpersonal relationships, happiness, having money and possessions, being healthy, pursuing work or school, achieving goals, being independent in ADL, and practicing religion or spirituality. The relative nature of life satisfaction was revealed by a respondent whose long-term care needs confined him to a wheelchair, that is, "life satisfaction is having my own wheelchair." He explained that wheelchairs in the institution were often uncomfortable and in need of repair, and that he was fortunate to own his own wheelchair. A man with quadriplegia expressed the pain of institutionalization in his description of life satisfaction, that is, "being able to live in my house, drive my car, and take care of my family."

People with long-term care needs included independence in ADL more frequently in their descriptions of both health and life satisfaction than did individuals without long-term care needs. Therefore, the lack of support for a relationship between power and perceived health in people with long-term care needs may be associated with their actual or perceived inability to independently perform ADL which, for them, characterizes health. Emphasis on independence in ADL by people with long-term care needs might also reflect the physical rehabilitation focus in the facility.

TRANSCENDENCE OF DISABILITY

Background questions were posed to ask participants whether or not religion and spirituality were important in their lives, and how often they engaged in prayer or meditation. Positive correlations were found between one or more of these variables and either power, health, or life satisfaction. Intercorrelations of importance of religion, importance of spirituality, and frequency of prayer or meditation in adults with long-term care needs may indicate that these variables are characteristics of an overall construct, transcendence, a manifestation of pandimensionality.

According to Rogers (1970), life has the capacity to transcend itself and to evolve toward greater diversity. Reed (1991) describes self-transcendence as "a pattern associated with advanced development that can occur in the context of a significant life event" (p. 71). Disability can be considered a significant life event associated with transcendence. Transcendence is a manifestation of the continuous mutual process of the pandimensional human-environmental energy fields, characterized by increasingly diverse patterns of religious beliefs and practices including spirituality, prayer, and meditation. Through religious or spiritual beliefs and practices, people with long-term care needs are able to transcend their arbitrary mind-body boundaries, participate in change, and experience awareness and well-being amid diverse patterns of health.

IMPLICATIONS

Researchers can utilize the findings of this study to develop a measure of well-being derived from the Science of Unitary Human Beings. Educators can teach appraisals of well-being that include clients' subjective reports of their health and life satisfaction. Practitioners can encourage people with long-term care needs to develop health-promoting behaviors as means for enhancing their power, health, and life satisfaction. Theorists may wish to further explore pandimensionality and the manifestation of transcendence, characterized by practices of religion, spirituality, prayer, and meditation, as it relates to power and well-being.

The current healthcare debate poses critical questions about what constitutes well-being, especially with regard to people with long-term care needs. These individuals are particularly vulnerable to service cutbacks in a climate of fiscal constraint, and may now have to compete with consumers of acute care services for dwindling healthcare dollars. As policymakers grapple with ethical dilemmas surrounding the reduction of services, people with long-term care needs face daily struggles with quality of life issues. At the crux of healthcare decisions are questions of choice, and the meaning of health and well-being. The research shows that people, including those with long-term care needs, participate knowingly in their well-being, and that well-being encompasses diverse pattern manifestations of health. Let our practice reflect the research as we respond to Rogers' (1992) charge "to promote health and well being for all persons wherever they are" (p. 28).

REFERENCES

Barrett, E. A. M. (1983). *An empirical investigation of Martha E. Rogers' principle of helicy: The relationship of human field motion and power.* Unpublished doctoral dissertation, New York University, New York. (University Microfilms No. 84-06278).

Barrett, E. A. M. (1990). Health patterning with clients in a private practice environment. In E. A. M. Barrett (Ed.), *Visions of Rogers' science-based nursing* (pp. 105–115). New York: NLN Press.

Brody, H., & Sobel, D. S. (1979). A systems view of health and disease. In D. S. Sobel (Ed.), *Ways of health: Holistic approaches to ancient and contemporary medicine* (pp. 87–104). New York: Harcourt Brace Jovanovich.

Campbell, A., Converse, P. E., & Rodgers, W. L. (1976). *The quality of American life: Perceptions, evaluations, and satisfactions.* New York: Russell Sage Foundation.

Cantril, H. (1965). *The pattern of human concerns.* New Brunswick, NJ: Rutgers University Press.

Conte, V. A., & Salamon, M. J. (1982). An objective approach to the measurement and use of life satisfaction with older persons *Measurement and Evaluation in Guidance, 15,*(3), 194–199.

Ference, H. M. (1979). *The relationship of time experience, creativity traits, differentiation, and human field motion.* Unpublished doctoral dissertation, New York University, New York. (University Microfilms No. 80-10281).

Ference, H. M. (1986). The relationship of time experience, creativity traits, differentiation, and human field motion. In V. M. Malinski (Ed.), *Explorations on Martha Rogers' science of unitary human beings* (pp. 95-116). Norwalk, CT: Appleton-Century-Crofts.

Fitzpatrick, J. J. (1983). A life perspective rhythm model. In J. J. Fitzpatrick & A. L. Whall (Eds.), *Conceptual models of nursing: Analysis and application* (pp. 295-302). Bowie, MD: Robert J. Brady.

Friedland, R. B. (1990). *Facing the costs of long-term care: An EBRI-ERF policy study.* Washington, DC: Employee Benefit Research Institute.

George, L. K., & Bearon, L. B. (1980). *Quality of life in older persons.* New York: Human Sciences Press.

Hunsberger, B. (1985). Religion, age, life satisfaction, and perceived sources of religiousness: A study of older persons. *Journal of Gerontology, 40*(5), 615-620.

Hurrelmann, K. (1989). *Human development and health.* Berlin, Germany: Springer-Verlag.

Jones, C. J. (1991). *Relationship of participation in health promotion behaviors to health-related hardiness and other selected factors in older adults.* Unpublished doctoral dissertation, Texas Woman's University, Dallas.

Levitt, M. J., Clark, M. C., Rotton, J., & Finley, G. E. (1987). Social support, perceived control, and well-being: A study of an environmentally stressed population. *International Journal of Aging and Human Development, 25*(4), 247-258.

Madrid, M., & Winstead-Fry, P. (1986). Rogers's conceptual model. In P. Winstead-Fry (Ed.), *Case studies in nursing theory* (pp. 73-102). New York: NLN Press.

Marx, K. (1970). The materialistic conception of history. In M. E. Olsen (Ed.), *Power in societies* (pp. 77-78). New York: Macmillan.

McNiff, M. A. (1996). A study of the relationship of power, perceived health, and life satisfaction in adults with long-term care needs based on Martha E. Rogers' science of unitary human beings. *Dissertation Abstracts International, 56*, 6037B.

Olsen, M. E. (Ed.). (1970). *Power in societies.* New York: Macmillan.

Parsons, T. (1979). Definitions of health and illness in the light of American values and social structure. In E. G. Jaco (Ed.), *Patients, physicians, and illness: A source book in behavioral science and health* (3rd ed., pp. 120-143). New York: Free Press.

Pope, A. M., & Tarlov, A. R. (Eds.). (1991). *Disability in America.* Washington, DC: National Academy Press.

Reed, P. G. (1987). Spirituality and well-being in terminally ill hospitalized adults. *Research in Nursing and Health, 10*, 335-344.

Reed, P. G. (1991). Toward a nursing theory of self-transcendence: Deductive reformulation using developmental theories. *Advances in Nursing Science, 13*(4), 64-77.

Rizzo, J. A. (1990). *An investigation of the relationships of life satisfaction, purpose in life, and power in persons sixty-five years and older.* Unpublished doctoral dissertation, New York University, New York.

Rogers, M. E. (1970). *An introduction to the theoretical basis of nursing.* Philadelphia: F.A. Davis.

Rogers, M. E. (1986). Science of unitary human beings. In V. M. Malinski (Ed.), *Explorations on Martha Rogers' science of unitary human beings* (pp. 3-8). Norwalk, CT: Appleton-Century-Crofts.

Rogers, M. E. (1990). Nursing: Science of unitary, irreducible, human beings: Update 1990. In E. A. M. Barrett (Ed.), *Visions of Rogers' science-based nursing* (pp. 5-11). New York: NLN Press.

Rogers, M. E. (1992). Nursing science and the space age. *Nursing Science Quarterly, 5*(1), 27-34.

Rotter, J. B. (1982). *The development and applications of social learning theory: Selected papers.* New York: Praeger.

Siegel, B. S. (1986). *Love, medicine & miracles: Lessons learned about self-healing from a surgeon's experience with exceptional patients.* New York: Harper & Row.

Sobel, D. S. (1979). Introduction. In D. S. Sobel (Ed.), *Ways of health: Holistic approaches to ancient and contemporary medicine* (pp. 3-11). New York: Harcourt Brace Jovanovich.

Spreitzer, E., & Snyder, E. E. (1974). Correlates of life satisfaction among the aged. *Journal of Gerontology, 29*(4), 454-458.

Weber, M. (1970). The types of authority and imperative co-ordination. In M. E. Olsen (Ed.), *Power in societies* (pp. 35-39). New York: Macmillan.

16

The Place of Transcendence in Nursing's Science of Unitary Human Beings: Theory and Research

Pamela G. Reed

*T*ranscendence is a disturbing word to many scientists, implying a realm that cannot be known scientifically, that is beyond the limits of knowledge and experience. Some may think it contradictory that the words transcendence and science are used together in the title of this chapter. On this contradiction one might agree, if "transcendence" referred to something ineffable, indescribable or immeasurable, for Rogers (1970, 1990) explained that science has a language of specificity that provides for precision, clarity, and communication, and in which testable hypotheses can be derived and research replicated.

In the nursing literature, the term "transcendence" has acquired more sophistication and more diversity in its meaning than as a lofty, incomprehensible concept, or a word that means simply to have climbed beyond. Sarter (1988) was one of the first scholars to call attention to the potential significance of the term as an underlying theme in the philosophical foundation of nursing's metaparadigm. Nursing theorists used the term to signify human processes critical to healing, transformation, human development, and well-being. Thus, it would seem that the concept of transcendence must have a place in nursing science. Transcendence as a scientific concept, can potentially become a part of what Rogers (1990) explained was the description, explanation and vision of science that strengthens nursing practice.

TRANSCENDENCE IN CLASSICAL NURSING THEORIES

Watson (1988), in her theory of human caring, described transcendence as integral to understanding the true nature of human beings as unbounded by temporal and spatial parameters, and as having inner strength. Transcendence meant an evolution toward spiritual levels of awareness that extended beyond the physical or material world. Watson (1988) regarded transcendence as more than a theoretical concept; it also signified a caring-healing context of the nurse and patient.

Parse (1992), in her theory of human becoming, used the term to refer to a set of paradoxical rhythmicities people engage in to move beyond the moment to forge new and unique ways of becoming. Powering, originating, and transforming are key verbs that describe the meaning of cotranscendence in human becoming theory. Transcendence is mobilized through true presence of the nurse and other person.

In Newman's (1995) theory of health as expanding consciousness, transcendence is a process by which the person confronts and moves beyond self-limitations toward a higher level of consciousness. Transcendence involves movement toward higher levels of complexity and creativity. Nurses facilitate transcendence by helping people translate observed patterns into an awareness of and fuller participation in their underlying pattern, which is unfolding in expanding consciousness.

Rogers (1990) was not as explicit nor did she write as much about the term transcendence as did other classical nursing theorists. She expressed the idea that it was the nature of life to transcend itself, and in her later years talked about a "transcendence unity" (Rogers, Doyle, Racolin, & Walsh, 1990). Her lack of elaboration about transcendence is an invitation, if not a challenge, for nurses to engage in dialogue about human transcendence to further develop the Science of Unitary Human Beings and to understand the nature of human evolution and its unpredictable potentialities. Rogers regarded science as an open process, open to new insights, new applications, new interpretations.

TRANSCENDENCE AND THE PRINCIPLES OF HOMEODYNAMICS

Rogers' (1990) three Principles of Homeodynamics are a useful guide for building ideas about the place of transcendence in the science. The principles address key questions about change in unitary human beings, relevant to understanding transcendence. Transcendence is a change process or pattern, and as such, functions in accord with the Principles of Homeodynamics.

Integrality

A first question to address in developing ideas about transcendence in the Science of Unitary Human Beings is "What is the *context* or setting of transcendence?" Or, more simply, "Just where does it take place and where does one look to study or facilitate it?" Rogers' (1990) Principle of Integrality indicates that pandimensionality is the context of change, manifested by a mutual process of person and environment.

This integrality-based view contrasts with physicalist ontology, whereby the context for health processes such as transcendence would be defined purely in terms of the observable body, no more and no less. Integrality also contrasts with 17th-century dualist thought, which posited a transcendental self separate from physical self, with the mind or act of thought being a necessary condition, as in Descartes' famous quotation, "I think, therefore I am." This view implies that there is a disembodied mind functioning separate from the body. Olafson (1995), a contemporary philosopher, stated that in dualism, every action, except those that were empirically observed by scientists, was withdrawn from the natural object itself and assigned to the mind. Last, integrality is incompatible with the interactionist paradigm of the mid-20th century, in which person and environment are regarded as separate but interacting systems. As Heidegger explained, human beings are not *in* the world, they *have* a world.

So, the context of transcendence cannot be embodied (as a cardiovascular system or synapse) nor disembodied (as a superego or mind, as higher consciousness or external environment); although each alone may be the focus of other scientists, these do not comprise the context of focus for Rogerian scientists and practitioners. Rogers' principle of integrality suggests, at the least, that transcendence takes place within a profound awareness of pandimensionality, in a context of mutuality among processes that, for lack of Rogerian terms have heretofore been described as inner-self and outer-self, and past, present, and future.

Helicy

A second question to address in building a Rogerian view of transcendence is "What is the nature of transcendence?" "How is it manifested?" A key characteristic of unitary human beings that has implications for understanding the nature of transcendence is the capacity to self-organize. Self-organizing is a term used across many theories—biologic and psychologic theories, chaos and complexity theories—to refer to a structure that changes in complexity and organization over time, and in so doing, gives way to qualitative change, whether it is a crystal, the boiling point of water, or a deeper understanding of a life event that emerges. In the context of nursing, this principle of self-organizing is represented in Rogers' (1980) Principle of Helicy, whereby the nature of change is described as "innovative and increasing diversity," and, also as "increasing complexification of energy field patterning" (Rogers, 1990, p. 8).

Open, living systems, such as human beings and human groups possess a natural tendency toward two kinds of change—diversity and innovation. Historically, other terms have been used to describe these changes. For example, in his seminal work on development, Werner (1957) explained this process as his "Orthogenetic Principle," which posited that living organisms change over time from lower to higher levels of both differentiation (also referred to as complexity or diversity) and integration (also referred to as nonlinear organization). Although various terms have been used to describe the self-organizing process, unitary patterning involves a mutuality of two ongoing processes, diversity and innovation.

Rhythmic patterning, in a person who is sick or well, means that increasing diversity is accompanied by innovation. Diversity without innovation is not rhythmic patterning, and instead is more of a chaotic patterning. Increasing diversity alone would become aimless and lack depth unless organized into meaningful experiences through innovation. And innovation without diversity would manifest as lacking breadth and richness, and as being narrow in perspective, highly specialized, and inflexible.

The innovation and diversity of transcendence, then, is manifested, for example, in persons with spinal cord injuries who develop different pathways that link together the diverse and shattered parts of life and bodily functions; in premature infants who manifest innovation as they organize the diversity of their person-environment process; and in older adults who reminisce as a way of making innovations out of the great diversity that has accumulated in their lives. Transcendence is evident in the healing after loss of a loved one or occurrence of chronic illness, which requires innovation and integration of many diverse experiences, including memories of the past, future dreams, altered rhythms and routines, pain and other chronic illness symptoms, sadness and self-doubt. In Sach's 1995 book, *An Anthropologist on Mars,* transcendence is depicted through stories about people with various maladies (e.g., colorblind painter, a surgeon with Tourette's syndrome) who were able to create a new organization that fit with their altered needs and world. These health events, in all their initial complexity and heartbreak gave rise to metamorphoses and innovation.

Resonancy

The third and final question to address in constructing a Rogerian view of transcendence is "Where is all this ongoing change going?" Rogers' (1980) Principle of Resonancy, as well as contemporary complexity theories (Kauffman, 1995), explain that despite the unpredictability of human change, there is pattern and purpose. The resonancy principle is quite clear that there is pattern in the ongoing change, represented in Rogers' (1990, 1992) words, "from lower to higher frequency wave patterns," with a purpose of fulfilling people's own rhythmicities.

So, unitary human beings are headed somewhere in change, and it is not primarily a change in quantity; it is qualitative, rhythmic change—the most basic definition of human development (Reed, 1983). Unlike mechanistic definitions of development that imply linear change in quantity, development more appropriately refers to a nonlinear process of *change in form,* as in the word, transformation. This is distinguished from growth, which refers to a *change in size.* The word, development, derives from the Old French word, "desvoloper," meaning to unwrap, unroll, or unfold, to realize basic potential through a nonadditive process of transformation. Human beings are profoundly developmental.

In other definitions of development that complement Rogers' resonancy principle are:

1. To set forth or make clear in degrees;
2. To elaborate by unfolding a musical idea by the working out of rhythmic and harmonic changes in the theme; and
3. To evolve the possibilities (Webster's, 1979).

The implications of Rogers' (1990) resonancy principle, then, is that unitary human beings are going somewhere, and that at least part of the journey is directed toward experiences of well-being that come from ful-filling one's own rhythmicities of changing diversity and innovation. This journey is not as linear or predictable as the words "from lower to higher frequency wave patterns" initially may imply; there are ups and downs, setbacks and leaps, tradeoffs and gains, and other rhythmicities, which one reaches to describe with these and other linear terms.

TRANSCENDENCE: SELF-ORGANIZING FOR WELL-BEING

Rogers' principles of homeodynamics taken as a whole reflect the basic capacity of unitary human beings, as individuals or groups, to self-organize for well-being. Transcendence represents one example of this ca-pacity of self-organizing for well-being.

Reed (1991a) studied transcendence as one example of self-organizing for well-being in later adulthood and during end-of-life experiences. More specifically, self-transcendence was regarded as a manifestation of a pat-tern of wholeness at times in life when a sense of fragmentation may threaten one's well-being. Self-transcendence refers to a fluctuation of per-ceived boundaries that extends the person (or self) beyond the immediate and constricted views of self and the world. This fluctuation is pandimen-sional, that is, outward (toward others and the environment), inward (to-ward greater awareness of one's own beliefs, values, and dreams), and temporal (toward integration of past and future in a way that enhances the relative present).

A key assumption underlying the study and measurement of self-transcendence is that an awareness of the integrality of self and world is an essential element in well-being. Human beings are open, pandimen-sional systems. They are capable of an awareness that extends beyond physical and temporal dimensions in rather ordinary ways, some of which are listed in Reed's (1991a) "Self-Transcendence Scale." In contrast to the more exotic images that the term may evoke, the "Self-Transcendence Scale" measures the terrestrial ways in which people reflect their inte-grality and integrate the complexities of life in a manner that is mediated by their everyday experiences (Gill, 1989).

A second assumption is that there is paradox in the awareness of one's pandimensionality. Kline (1995) describes this paradox in terms of peo-ple being unbounded in their openness to the world, yet ontologically closed by the visible substances that make up the world. Rogers (1970) stated that "the human field is characterized by continuously fluctuating imaginary boundaries" (pp. 331–332). Self-transcendence, as derived from Rogerian ontology, is a profound awareness of fluctuating bound-aries that are grounded in, yet reach beyond, the temporal and terrestrial

(Reed, 1995). Human beings characteristically impose perceived or conceptual boundaries on their openness to define their reality and provide a sense of connectedness and wholeness.

Reed's (1989, 1991a) research on self-transcendence was based on the theoretical idea that there is an important relationship between fluctuations of imaginary boundaries and well-being across the lifespan and health experiences. Self-boundaries fluctuate over time in patterns of diversity and innovation, and correlate with various indicators of well-being. In constructing her middle-range theory, Reed (1991b) regarded self-transcendence as a resource that emerges out of health experiences that confront the person with personal mortality/immortality, as found in life-threatening illness, advanced age, and chronic illness, for example. Self-transcendence is evoked by these events in a way that allows the person to integrate the disparate, complex, and conflicting elements of living, aging, and dying. Critical health events confront people with diversity, in terms of people, new experiences, information, fears and other feelings, which they then must organize into some meaningful package for well-being to occur.

Self-transcendence is not merely a nice resource to have during critical health events or in later life; it is a natural resource for healing that manifests the human being's capacity to self-organize for well-being. Self-transcendence may be viewed as a homeodynamic imperative, meaning that it is a human resource that emerges as part of the life process and it demands participation on the person's part in order to maintain well-being during a given life situation. Other examples of homeodynamic imperatives are grieving in bereaved persons, toddlers walking, and anxiety in persons faced with new situations. One wouldn't dream of curtailing a toddler's practice of walking or a bereaved person's grieving process. Similarly, self-transcendence may be an important form of expression during illness or other potentially fragmenting experiences.

Empirical findings generated through both qualitative and quantitative research methods indicate that inadequate expressions of, or opportunities for, self-transcendence contribute to health experiences and diminished well-being. Transcendence is not only a capacity, but a participatory process and a struggle, as attested to, for example, by survivors of breast cancer (Coward & Reed, 1996). A sample of the findings from research over the past decade indicates that self-transcendence is integral to well-being in a variety of health experiences that confront one with end-of-life issues. Self-transcendence has been found to be related to: diminished clinical depression (Reed, 1986, 1989, 1991a); diminished loneliness in older adults (Walton, Shultz, Beck, & Walls, 1991); well-being in women with end-stage breast cancer (Coward, 1990, 1991); well-being in gay men and women with AIDS (Coward & Lewis, 1993; Coward, 1995); diminished suicidality in geriatric hospitalized patients (Buchanan, Farran, & Clark, 1995); greater will to live and diminished depression in psychiatric out-patients (Reed & McGaffic, 1994); increased hopefulness and care of oneself in chronically ill elders in home health care (Reed, 1992); greater complexity and integration in moral reasoning about end-of-life dilemmas in elders (Reed, Mezza, & Jacobs, 1996); and successful psychotherapy among elder group therapy patients (Young & Reed, 1995).

Poet and research participant Wahnita DeLong published a poem (circa 1980), titled "After Ninety." The poem eloquently expresses her experience of self-transcendence at the end of life. She has since passed on, but her poem remains to convey in words DeLong's fulfilling of her own rhythmicities:

After Ninety

(Dedicated to the memory of Martha Rogers)

> *Now you have come to the time*
> *when you can feel*
> *the shape of things to come*
> *mystic, real;*
>
> *Now you can see*
> *you are a part of all*
> *that ever was*
> *of all that is to be;*
>
> *Now you know*
> *you had no day of birth*
> *you cannot die,*
> *you walk the earth*
> *but your reach is the sky;*
>
> *Now where you are*
> *you have become the essence*
> *of root and star.*

DeLong, circa 1980

REFERENCES

Buchanan, D., Farran, C., & Clark, D. (1995). Suicidal thought and self-transcendence in older adults. *Journal of Psychosocial Nursing, 33*(10), 31-34.

Coward, D. (1990). The lived experience of self-transcendence in women with advanced breast cancer. *Nursing Science Quarterly, 3,* 162–169.

Coward, D. (1995). Lived experience of self-transcendence in women with AIDS. *Journal of Obstetrics, Gynecology and Neonatal Nursing, 24,* 314–338.

Coward, D., & Lewis, F. (1993). The lived experience of self-transcendence in gay men with AIDS. *Oncology Nursing Forum, 20,* 1363–1369.

Coward, D., & Reed, P. G. (1996). Self-transcendence: A resource for healing at the end of life. *Issues in Mental Health Nursing, 17,* 275–288.

DeLong, W. (circa 1980). After Ninety. In *Other places, other times.* Evansville, IN: Whipperwill.

Gill, J. H. (1989). *Mediated transcendence: A postmodern reflection.* Macon, GA: Mercer University Press.

Kauffman, S. (1995). *At home in the universe: The search for laws of self-organization and complexity.* New York: Oxford University Press.

Kline, S. J. (1995). *Conceptual foundations for multidisciplinary thinking.* Stanford, CA: Stanford University Press.

Newman, M. (1995). *Health as expanding consciousness (2nd ed.).* New York: NLN Press.

Olafson, F. A. (1995). *What is a human being? A Heideggerian view.* New York: Cambridge University Press.

Parse, R. R. (1992). Human becoming: Parse's theory of nursing. *Nursing Science Quarterly, 5*(1), 35–42.

Reed, P. G. (1983). Implications of the life-span developmental framework for well-being in adulthood and aging. *Advances in Nursing Science, 6*(1), 18–25.

Reed, P. G. (1986). Developmental resources and depression in the elderly: A longitudinal study. *Nursing Research, 35,* 368–374.

Reed, P. G. (1989). Mental health of older adults. *Western Journal of Nursing Research, 11*(2), 143–163.

Reed, P. G. (1991a). Self-transcendence and mental health in oldest-old adults. *Nursing Research, 40*(1), 5–11.

Reed, P. G. (1991b). Toward a nursing theory of self-transcendence: Deductive reformulation using developmental theories. *Advances in Nursing Science, 13*(4), 64–77.

Reed, P. G. (1992). *Self-neglect in chronically ill elderly: Conceptual, empirical, and ethical dimensions.* Paper presented at the ANA Council of Nursing Researchers' International Conference, Los Angeles.

Reed, P. G. (1995). Transcendence: Formulating nursing perspectives. *Nursing Science Quarterly, 9*(1), 2–4.

Reed, P. G. & McGaffic, C. M. (1994). *Postformal reasoning as a mental health resource in later life.* Paper presented at the Western Society for Research in Nursing Conference, Phoenix, AZ.

Reed, P. G., Mezza, I., & Jacobs, M. (1996). *Elders' moral reasoning about end-of-life dilemmas.* Paper presented at the 23rd Nursing Research Conference, University of Arizona College of Nursing and Sigma Theta Tau Beta Mu Chapter, Rio Rico, AZ.

Rogers, M. E. (1970). *Introduction to the theoretical basis of nursing.* Philadelphia: F.A. Davis.

Rogers, M. E. (1980). A science of unitary man. In J. P. Riehl & C. Roy (Eds), *Conceptual models for nursing practice* (2nd ed.) pp. 329-337. New York: Appleton-Century-Crofts.

Rogers, M. E. (1990). Nursing: Science of unitary, irreducible, human beings: Update 1990. In E. A. M. Barrett (Ed.), *Visions of Rogers' science-based nursing* (pp. 5-12). New York: NLN Press.

Rogers, M. E. (1992). Nursing science and the space age. *Nursing Science Quarterly, 5*(1), 27-34.

Rogers, M. E., Doyle, M. B., Racolin, A., & Walsh, P. C. (1990). A conversation with Martha Rogers on nursing in space. In E. A. M. Barrett (Ed.), *Visions of Rogers' science-based nursing* (pp. 375-386). New York: NLN Press.

Sachs, O. (1995). *An anthropologist on Mars: Seven paradoxical tales.* New York: Knopf.

Sarter, B. (1988). Philosophical sources of nursing theory. *Nursing Science Quarterly, 1*(2), 52-59.

Walton, C. G., Shultz, C. M., Beck, C. M., & Walls, R. C. (1991). Psychological correlates of loneliness in the older adult. *Archives of Psychiatric Nursing, 5*(3), 165-170.

Watson, J. (1988). New dimensions of human caring theory. *Nursing Science Quarterly, 1,* 175-181.

Webster's New Collegiate Dictionary. (1979). Springfield, MA: G. & C. Merriam Co.

Werner, H. (1957). The concept of development from a comparative and organismic point of view. In D. B. Harris (Ed.), *The concept of development* (pp. 125-148). Minneapolis: University of Minnesota Press.

Young, C., & Reed, P. G. (1995). Elders' perceptions of the role of group psychotherapy in fostering self-transcendence. *Archives of Psychiatric Nursing, 9*(6), 338-347.

17

The Relationship of Temporal Experience and Power as Knowing Participation in Change in Depressed and Nondepressed Women

Violet M. Malinski

*D*epression is an issue of some importance in women's health. With women twice as likely as men to be diagnosed with unipolar depression (McGrath, Keita, Strickland, & Russo, 1990; Public Health Service Task Force on Women's Health Issues, 1985), it is estimated that 1 out of 10 women will experience severe depression at some point in the life span

The author gratefully acknowledges the assistance of Irving Bernstein, PhD, independent statistical consultant, and Ilene Wiletz, PhD, statistician with the Department of Grants Management and Research Support, Beth Israel Hospital. Thanks are extended to Elizabeth A. M. Barrett, RN; PhD, FAAN, for her critique of an earlier draft of this paper. This study was funded by a PSC-CUNY grant, Hunter College/CUNY.

(Weissman & Klerman, 1979). Characteristics of depression can include feelings of despondency, dejection, hopelessness, and helplessness; social withdrawal; psychomotor retardation; sleep disturbances; inability to mobilize the self; and suicidal thoughts (Haber, 1992).

From the perspective of Rogerian nursing science (Rogers, 1992), such characteristics can also be described as lower frequency field patterning. According to Rogers (1992), lower frequency patterns in the human/environmental field process include slower motion, time experienced as slower, and lesser diversity, whereas higher frequency field patterning includes faster motion, time experienced as faster to experiences of timelessness, and greater diversity. Characteristics of lower frequency patterning seem to describe the experience commonly called depression.

In this study, I sought to determine the relationship of temporal experience and power in depressed and nondepressed women. Given the similarities between descriptions of depression and examples of lower frequency field patterning, the relationships of these variables (temporal experience and power) that describe lower and higher frequency patterning phenomena were tested. The study was designed to test the following hypotheses:

1. The frequency of temporal experience, as measured by the three Temporal Experience Scales of Time Dragging, Time Racing, and Timelessness, is related to the frequency of power as measured by the four Power as Knowing Participation in Change concepts, awareness, choices, freedom to act intentionally, and involvement in creating changes.

2. Lower frequency temporal experience, as measured by the three Temporal Experience Scales of Time Dragging, Time Racing, and Timelessness, is related to lower frequency power as measured by the four Power as Knowing Participation in Change concepts, awareness, choices, freedom to act intentionally, and involvement in creating changes in depressed women.

3. Higher frequency temporal experience, as measured by the three Temporal Experience Scales of Time Dragging, Time Racing, and Timelessnessis related to higher frequency power as measured by the four Power as Knowing Participation in Change concepts, awareness, choices, freedom to act intentionally, and involvement in creating changes in nondepressed women.

4. Lower frequency temporal experience is related to higher depression scores.

5. Lower frequency power is related to higher depression scores.

THEORETICAL FRAMEWORK

Rogers' (1992) Science of Unitary Human Beings provides a framework for the present study. In this light, human and environment are irreducible, pandimensional energy fields identified by wave patterning that flows in lower and higher frequencies, continuously moving and changing. The principle of integrality describes the continuous mutual process of human and environmental fields. The principles of resonancy and helicy capture the flow or process of change (lower and higher frequencies) and the nature of change (increasing diversity).

Knowing participation in change has long been an assumption in Rogerian science. Change is seen as continuous and therefore cannot be started or stopped. What people can do is change the nature of their participation in that change process. Barrett (1986) has identified this knowing participation in change as power, developing a theory of power and a tool to measure it. She derived the power theory from the principle of helicy, operationalizing the field manifestations of power as awareness, choices, freedom to act intentionally, and involvement in creating changes. "Power is being aware of what one is choosing to do, feeling free to do it, and doing it intentionally" (Barrett, 1990, p. 108). This means participating in the process of change to actualize some potentials over others (higher frequency power). Lower frequency power, manifested by inhibited awareness, choices, freedom, and involvement, would seem to characterize the person experiencing depression. Indeed, feeling powerless is one potential characteristic of depression (Haber, 1992). McGrath (1992) offered the opinion that awareness and action are needed to convert "bad feelings . . . into new sources of energy, growth, creativity, and power" (p. 23) for depressed women.

Temporal experience is another manifestation of the relative diversity of human-environmental field patterning (Rogers, 1992). In depression, the subjective experience of time diminishes (Newman & Guadiano, 1984). Using Rogerian nursing science, Paletta (1990) developed the Temporal Experience Scales to capture the rhythmic flow of time, experienced as time passing. The three scales reflect the experiences of time dragging, the least diverse pattern manifestation; time racing, more diverse; and timelessness, the most diverse. The metaphors selected reflect lower to higher frequency patterning, for example, items suggesting little or no sense of movement, rapid movement, and motion experienced as a continuous flow.

METHOD

Participants

The volunteer sample was delimited to women ages 25 through 44, the age range within which three times as many women as men are treated for depression in outpatient settings (Bell & Goldman, 1980). Participants were recruited from the private practices of psychiatric-mental health nursing clinical specialists and feminist therapists from other disciplines in a large metropolitan area as well as from among students and colleagues in the researcher's academic setting. Snowball sampling was used. Following recommendations for minimum sample sizes of 200 for canonical correlation (Kerlinger & Pedhazur, 1973; Waltz & Bausell, 1981), 400 participants were obtained. The researcher continued collecting data until 200 sets of usable data were obtained in each group, a period of 2.5 years.

The depressed group had more married women with children, who had a college or high school education, worked either part-time or not at all, and had experienced more frequent negative life events. The nondepressed group had more single women without children, who had a college or graduate school education and worked full-time.

Instruments

Data collection tools consisted of Barrett's power tool, Paletta's Temporal Experience Scales, Beck's Depression Inventory, and a demographic data sheet. Permission for use was obtained for each tool.

The Beck Depression Inventory (Beck, 1972; Beck & Beck, 1972) was used to validate the diagnosis. It consists of 21 items reflecting symptoms and attitudes in the areas of mood alterations, negative self-concept, regressive and self-punitive wishes, vegetative symptoms, and changes in activity level. The range of possible scores is 0–63, with 0–9 reflecting the normal range, 10–15 mild depression, 16–19 mild-moderate, 20–29 moderate-severe, and 30–63 severe depression. In the sample of depressed women 45 (23%) scored as mildly to moderately depressed and 155 (77%) as mildly depressed. Reliability (split-half, internal consistency) and validity (construct and concurrent) have been established (Beck, 1972). In this study Cronbach's alpha reliability of .92 was obtained.

Barrett's (1986) Power as Knowing Participation in Change tool consists of four concepts or field behaviors (awareness, choices, freedom to act intentionally, and involvement in creating changes) measured by 52 semantic differential scales, 12 per concept and one each for re-test. Each adjective pair contains one higher frequency and one lower frequency choice. The tool was constructed following recommendations from two panels of judges knowledgeable in Rogerian nursing science and/or psycometric testing. Barrett pilot-tested it with a national sample of 267 women and men ages 19–60 and used factor analysis to select the items for a revised instrument. In the main study she obtained a volunteer national sample of 625 women and men, ages 21–60, representing a diverse group in terms of such variables as marital status, education, and occupation. Validity coefficients as determined by factor loadings for the concept-context measures of power ranged from 0.56 to 0.70, and reliabilities ranged from 0.63 to 0.99 (Barrett, 1986). The tool has been used in a variety of nursing studies (Bramlett & Gueldner, 1993; Caroselli, 1992; Dzurec, 1994; Kilker, 1994; Rapacz, 1991; Smith, 1994) with reliabilities ranging from .57 to .99. Alpha reliabilities obtained in this study were .89 for awareness, .90 for choices, .91 for freedom, and .92 for involvement, with a total power reliability of .97.

Paletta's (1990) Temporal Experience Scales reflect temporal perception time as time passing, evolving "through a lifetime of continuous mutual processes, culminating in the individual's current pattern of time sense in relation to the environment" (p. 241). Three independent 8-item Likert scales, Time Dragging, Time Racing, and Timelessness, reflect these patterns of temporal experience. In the instrument development sample, consisting of 305 men and women of various occupations, alpha reliabilities of .82, .74, and .79 respectively were obtained (Paletta, 1990). In a sample of 120 graduate students in nursing, women ages 20 through 40, reliabilities were .38, .72, and .74 respectively. In this study reliabilities of .87, .94, and .74 were obtained.

Procedure

The procedures and tools were approved prior to data collection by the college committee for the protection of human subjects. Data collection packets were distributed or mailed to the therapists who had agreed to ask clients if they were willing to participate and to colleagues and students. Extra packets were provided for those who offered to distribute them to other potential participants. Stamped, self-addressed envelopes were provided. Return of completed packets constituted consent to participate. No names or other identifying data were included.

A correlational design was employed, using canonical correlation as the data analysis method. Canonical correlation is an extension of multiple regression to two or more independent variables and two or more dependent ones. It specifies relations among sets of variables with tests of their significance (Duntemann, 1984; Kerlinger & Pedhazur, 1973). The procedure produces canonical variates, factors that share the maximum amount of variance between the sets of variables, for examination (Waltz & Bausell, 1981). Canonical correlation is appropriate when the first set of measures reflects one construct and the second set reflects a related construct (Kerlinger & Pedhazur, 1973), in this case temporal experience and power as manifestations of higher and lower frequency field diversity. The focus of the canonical correlation procedure on assessing relationships rather than predicting outcomes (Munro, 1986) is also consistent with the theoretical framework of this study.

The maximum number of canonical correlations cannot exceed the number in the smaller set of variables, in this case, three. The first canonical correlation reflects the highest possible correlation of linear combinations of each set, the second the next highest, and so on (Munro, 1986).

Results

Using SPSS-X, canonical correlation was performed within MANCOVA (SPSS-X User's Guide, 1988). The four power concepts (awareness, choices, freedom, and involvement) were treated as dependent variables with the three time scales (dragging, racing, and timelessness) as independent ones across the total sample and then in the depressed and nondepressed groups. Findings are presented in Table 17.1.

The first hypothesis was supported. In the overall sample, the first and second canonical variates had significant correlations, .539, $p < .0005$ and .210, $p = .002$, respectively. The combined R_c^2 of .331 accounted for 33 percent of the variance. An eigenvalue of .40 and above is considered excellent, while those approaching 0 are considered worthless (Hedderson & Fisher, 1993). Only one eigenvalue was significant, that for the first factor in the total sample (.409). Time Dragging (lower frequency temporal experience) was inversely related to awareness, choice, freedom, and involvement. Time Racing and the power concepts varied in the same direction.

Next a dimension reduction or redundancy analysis was performed. This shows patterns of correlations among the original variables and the canonical variates (Duntemann, 1984). The higher the redundancy, the better the predictive ability from one set of variables to the other (Munro, 1986). A value of "0" for Wilks lambda indicates that the independent variables account for all of the variance in the dependent variables while a value of "1" indicates that they account for none of the variance. The dimension reduction analysis (Wilks lambda = .674, $p < .001$) for the total sample showed that three functions together accounted for 33 percent of the variance,

Table 17.1   Canonical Correlations of Temporal Experience and Power

Canonical Correlations	Variables			
	Temporal Experience		Power	
	Entire Sample ($N = 400$)			
First	Dragging	.954*	Awareness	−.886
$R_c = .539$	Racing	−.938	Choice	−.970
$p < .0005$	Timelessness	−.308	Freedom	−.777
$R_c^2 = .291$			Involvement	−.821
Second	Timelessness	.949	Involvement	−.324
$R_c = .210$				
$p = .002$				
$R_c^2 = .04$				
	Depressed Sample ($N = 200$)			
First	Racing	−.943	Freedom	.678
$R_c = .306$			Involvement	.832
$p = .012$				
$R_c^2 = .094$				
	Nondepressed Sample ($N = 200$)			
First	Dragging	−.771	Awareness	.775
$R_c = .313$	Racing	.784	Choice	.611
$p = .005$	Timelessness	−.700	Freedom	.643
$R_c^2 = .098$			Involvement	.88

*Only correlations at or above .30, the cutoff for significance (Pedazur, 1982), are reported.

with the first function accounting for 28 percent of that variance, similar to the squared canonical correlation yielding 29 percent. Therefore, the first function alone is probably sufficient (SPSS, 1988). The Roy-Bargman Stepdown F test demonstrated that awareness, choices, and involvement contributed to statistically significant ($p < .001$) association with the set of temporal variables while freedom ($p = .468$) did not.

Regarding hypotheses two and three, in the depressed and nondepressed groups the canonical correlations for the first variates achieved significance, .306, $p = .012$ and .313, $p = .005$, respectively. However, the corresponding eigenvalues were not significant (.103 and .109) and the Wilks lambda values were high (.842, about 16% of the variance, and .867, 13%), so they must be examined with caution. The trends for association seem to reflect an inverse relationship between time racing and freedom and involvement in the depressed sample and a positive correlation between time racing and awareness, choices, freedom, and involvement in the nondepressed sample. In general, to the extent that one experiences time as dragging, one also experiences diminished awareness, choices, freedom, and involvement.

For hypotheses four and five, one-way analyses of variance were conducted to explore how the time and power scales varied according to the depression categories of normal, mildly depressed, and mildly to moderately depressed. The nondepressed group had significantly different ($p < .05$) temporal (racing) and power (higher frequency) scale values than the depressed group. There was no significant difference in the two categories of depression on these scale values.

Supplemental Analyses

Pearson correlations were computed to measure the strength of relationships among the power, time, and depression scales. Scores on the Beck Depression Inventory correlated positively with time dragging ($r = .82$, $p < .001$) and negatively with time racing ($r = -.83, p < .001$) and timelessness ($r = -.33, p < .001$). Depression correlated negatively with the overall power scale ($r = -.53, p < .001$) and with the four subscales (awareness, $r = -.47, p < .001$; choice, $r = -.54, p < .001$; freedom, $r = -.43, p < .001$; involvement, $r = -46, p < .001$). The power subscales intercorrelated highly with each other and with the overall scale.

Multiple regression analysis was performed to examine how time and power related to depression scale values. Variables were entered sequentially in a stepwise regression, and the proportion of variance was adjusted each time a new variable was added to the equation. The first equation showed that the three temporal scales and the choice subscale of the power tool accounted for nearly 78 percent of the variance in depression values. Again, time racing had a strong negative correlation with depression (Beta $= -.83$) whereas time dragging showed a positive correlation (Beta $= .42$). Timelessness and choices showed low but significant ($p < .001$) negative correlations with depression (Beta $= -.12$ and $-.12$ respectively). Awareness, freedom, and involvement fell out of the equation as not significant.

The second equation examined the power scale alone in relation to depression. Choice and involvement were retained as predictive, accounting for about 32 percent of the variance. Awareness and freedom accounted for only 7 percent of the variance.

The third equation examined the temporal scale alone in relation to depression. All three subscales were retained as predictive, accounting for 77 percent of the variance in depression. Again, there is a strong negative correlation between time racing and depression.

DISCUSSION

The analysis suggested a relationship between temporal experience and power in depressed and nondepressed women that is reflected in diversity of pattern. Lower frequency, less diverse temporal experience (dragging) is related to lower frequency, less diverse power. Higher frequency, greater diversity of temporal experience (racing) is related to higher frequency manifestations of power. The temporal pattern postulated to be the most diverse, timelessness, was not readily manifested in this sample. Paletta (1990) noted that temporal development proceeds with the experience of movement, from the perception of slow movement (dragging) through racing and timelessness. The latter is the experience of being one with the universe, integral with the flow of time, rather than the perception of "life events as moving past one" (Paletta, 1990, p. 240).

What is particularly striking, given the high proportion of individuals scoring mildly depressed and the lack of individuals scoring as moderately to severely and severely depressed on the Beck scale, is the strong relationship between time dragging and depression. Theoretically this makes sense; it mirrors the experience of depression as one of being stuck, feeling sluggish, going nowhere. In Paletta's (1990) sample of volunteer female graduate students in nursing, Time Dragging and Time Racing were correlated; the regression analysis "neither supported nor refuted the direction and magnitude" of these scales (p. 248). In the current study, individuals clearly manifested differences in temporal experience according to dragging and racing.

Regarding the lack of depression scores reflecting moderate and severe depression, it is possible that the depressed individuals, all currently in treatment, wished to appear less depressed and answered the Beck accordingly. No attempt was made in this study to ascertain prior exposure to this tool or to correlate depression scores with either clinical assessments of severity or length of treatment. This would be worth exploring in future studies. Moving to inpatient psychiatric settings could provide access to a population more severely depressed than an outpatient group. Although a sample of 200 is given as the minimum for canonical correlation, the mixed findings in the correlation analysis for the depressed and nondepressed groups suggest the need for larger numbers.

It would be interesting to identify pattern profiles of individuals diagnosed as depressed using a range of quantitative measurement tools developed in Rogerian nursing science. In addition to the power tool and Temporal Experience Scales used in this study, other tools such as Human Field Motion (Ference, 1986), the Index of Field Energy (Gueldner, 1993), the Diversity of Human Field Pattern Scale (Hastings-Tolsma, 1994), the

Human Field Image Metaphor Scale (Johnston, 1994), and the Person-Environment Participation Scale (Leddy, 1995) could be used to assemble such pattern profiles. Barrett (1986) correlated the power tool with Human Field Motion, finding a relationship of higher frequency power and accelerated human field motion. Rapacz (1991) found that a group experiencing chronic pain manifested lower frequency field patterning as measured by Human Field Motion and Power. Pattern profiles assembled by such quantitative tools could be compared with qualitative pattern profile methods, such as Carboni's (1992) Mutual Exploration of the Healing Human Field-Environmental Field Relationship and Butcher's (1995) Unitary Field Pattern Portrait Research Method.

Using the latter, Butcher (1995) was able to identify a phenomenon that he saw as distinct from the medical diagnosis of depression. Looking at "dispiritedness" in later life, he identified such themes as dissipating energy, loneliness, disconnectedness, dwindling vitality, and declining will to live. Simultaneously, Butcher (1995) identified the rhythm of inspiritedness, "accelerating movement toward patterns of greater diversity manifested by visioning infinite potentials and creating innovative ways of actively participating in the later life process" (p. 3). Together, dispiritedness-inspiritedness forms a continuous rhythm.

Rogers' suggested manifestations of change can be seen as continuous rhythms. (Rogers tried to move away from suggestions of linearity in these manifestations by deleting the language of "from . . . to"). The continuous rhythm of temporal experience, for example, can be seen as flowing in lower and higher frequencies, with the experiences of dragging, racing, and timelessness as human-environmental field potentials being actualized throughout the life process. The second (nonsignificant) variate for the depressed group disclosed a relationship among dragging, timelessness, freedom, and involvement. This accounted for only 6 percent of the variance and had a significance level of .09, but it may disclose a trend that could become clearer with a larger sample, suggesting this type of continuous rhythm.

The findings have implications for nursing practice. Nurses may be the first healthcare professionals to detect signs of depression in clients. Rogerian nursing practice begins with the energy field pattern and ways to appraise it through experiences, perceptions, and expressions that manifest the pattern (Cowling, 1990). Barrett (1990) has outlined a practice methodology based on pattern manifestation appraisal and deliberative mutual patterning. The power tool and Temporal Experience Scales can be used in pattern appraisal. By mutually exploring manifestations of pattern, nurse and client together can knowingly participate in the health patterning process. Therapeutic touch, imagery, meditation, laughter and humor, light and color, music and movement, personal narrative and storytelling, and journaling are some examples of health patterning modalities that can be explored in future research for their potential to expand the range of choices available to those diagnosed as depressed.

REFERENCES

Barrett, E. A. M. (1986). Investigation of the principle of helicy: The relationship of human field motion and power. In V. M. Malinski (Ed.), *Explorations on Martha Rogers' science of unitary human beings* (pp. 173–184). Norwalk, CT: Appleton-Century-Crofts.

Barrett, E. A. M. (1990). Rogers' science-based nursing practice. In E. A. M. Barrett (Ed.), *Visions of Rogers' science-based nursing* (pp. 31–44). New York: NLN Press.

Beck, A. T. (1972). *Depression: Causes and treatments.* Philadelphia: University of Pennsylvania.

Beck, A. T., & Beck, R. W. (1972). Screening depressed patients in family practice: A rapid screening technique. *Postgraduate Medicine, 56*(6), 81–85.

Belle, D., & Goldman, N. (1980). Patterns of diagnoses received by men and women. In M. Guttentgag, S. Salasin, & D. Belle (Eds.), *The mental health of women* (pp. 21–30). New York: Academic Press.

Bramlett, M. H., & Gueldner, S. H. (1993). Reminiscence: A viable option to enhance power in elders. *Clinical Nurse Specialist, 7,* 60–74.

Butcher, H. K. (1995). A unitary field pattern portrait of dispiritedness in later life [Abstract]. *Rogerian Nursing Science News, 7*(3), 1–2.

Carboni, J. T. (1992). Instrument development and the measurement of unitary constructs. *Nursing Science Quarterly, 5,* 134–142.

Caroselli, C. (1992). The relationship of power and feminism in female nurse executives in acute care hospitals [Abstract]. *Rogerian Nursing Science News, 5*(1), 3–4.

Cowling, W. R. (1990). A template for unitary pattern-based practice. In E. A. M. Barrett (Ed.), *Visions of Rogers' science-based nursing practice* (pp. 45–65). New York: NLN Press.

Duntemann, G. H. (1984). *Introduction to multivariate analysis.* Beverly Hills, CA: Sage.

Dzurec, L. (1994). Schizophrenic clients' experiences of power: Using hermeneutic analysis. *Image: The Journal of Nursing Scholarship, 5,* 155–159.

Ference, H. M. (1986). The relationship of time experience, creativity traits, differentiation, and human field motion. In V. M. Malinski (Ed.), *Explorations on Martha Rogers' science of unitary human beings* (pp. 95–105). Norwalk, CT: Appleton-Century-Crofts.

Gueldner, S. H. (1993). *A psychometric analysis of the index of human field energy.* Unpublished manuscript.

Haber, J. (1992). Management of suicide and depression. In J. Haber, A. L. McMahon, P. Price-Hoskins, & B. F. Sideleau (Eds.), *Comprehensive psychiatric nursing* (4th ed., pp. 549–581). St. Louis, MO: Mosby.

Hastings-Tolsma, M. T. (1994). The relationship of diversity of human field pattern to risk-taking and time experience: An investigation of Rogers' principles of homeodynamics [Abstract]. *Rogerian Nursing Science News, 6*(4), 6-7.

Hedderson, J., & Fisher, M. (1993). *SPSS made simple* (2nd ed). Belmont, CA: Wadsworth.

Johnston, L. W. (1994). Psychometric analysis of Johnston's human field image metaphor scale. *Visions: The Journal of Rogerian Nursing Science, 2,* 7-11.

Kerlinger, F. N., & Pedhazur, E. J. (1973). *Multiple regression in behavioral research.* New York: Holt, Rinehart and Winston.

Kilker, M. J. (1994). Transformational and transactional leadership styles: An empirical investigation of Rogers' principle of integrality [Abstract]. *Rogerian Nursing Science News, 7*(2), 1.

Leddy, S. K. (1995). Measuring mutual process: Development and psychometric testing of the person-environment participation scale. *Visions: The Journal of Rogerian Nursing Science, 3,* 20-31.

McGrath, E. (1992). *When feeling bad is good.* New York: Holt.

McGrath, E., Keita, G. P., Strickland, B. R., & Russo, N. F. (1990). *Women and depression: Risk factors and treatment issues.* Washington, DC: American Psychological Association.

Munro, B. H. (1986). Canonical correlation and discriminant function analysis. In B. H. Munro, M. A. Visintainer, & E. B. Page (Eds.), *Statistical methods for health care research* (pp. 320-333). Philadelphia: Lippincott.

Newman, M. A., & Guadiano, J. K. (1984). Depression as an explanation for decreased subjective time in the elderly. *Nursing Research, 33,* 137-139.

Paletta, J. L. (1990). The relationship of temporal experience to human time. In E. A. M. Barrett (Ed.), *Visions of Rogers' science-based nursing* (pp. 239-252). New York: NLN Press.

Pedhazur, E. J. (1982). *Multiple regression in behavioral research* (2nd ed.). New York: Holt, Rinehart and Winston.

Public Health Service Task Force on Women's Health Issues. (1985). Women's health: Report of the Public Health Service Task Force on Women's Issues. *Public Health Reports, 100*(1), 73-106.

Rapacz, K. E. (1991). Human patterning and chronic pain [Abstract]. *Rogerian Nursing Science News, 4*(1), 1-2.

Rogers, M. E. (1992). Nursing science and the space age. *Nursing Science Quarterly, 5,* 27-34.

Smith, D. W. (1994). Toward developing a theory of spirituality. *Visions: The Journal of Rogerian Nursing Science, 2,* 35-43.

SPSS-X user's guide (3rd ed.) (1988). Chicago: SPSS.

Waltz, C., & Bausell, R. B. (1981). *Nursing research: Designs, statistics, and computer analysis.* Philadelphia: F.A. Davis.

Weissman, M. N., & Klerman, G. L. (1979). Sex differences and the etiology of depression. In E. S. Gomberg & V. Franks (Eds.), *Gender and disordered behavior.* New York: Brunner/Mazel.

Part Five

Patterns of Rogerian Knowing in Practice

18

The Pandimensional
Nurse Manager

Bela Horvath

*I*n a scene from the classic film "The Graduate," a bewildered-looking Dustin Hoffman is approached at a wedding party by a business associate of the family who offers some unsolicited career advice. "PLASTIC" intones the well-intended but over-zealous advisor; the implication being that his future success would be all but guaranteed by delving into the plastics market.

My own ascendence into nursing management evolved through similar scenarios, as it seemed that nearly everyone I spoke with had an opinion on how to shape my career. At the time (the early 1980s), the prevalent opinion was for me, being a baccalaureate-prepared *male* nurse, to get an MBA. Some recommended I pursue an MPH. Many of my peers suggested I leave nursing altogether and study psychology or social work for continued upward mobility.

I returned to my alma mater (NYU) to pursue a graduate degree in the Delivery of Nursing Service. There, my understanding of and insights into Martha Rogers' conceptual system grew deeper, and the potential applications to my work as a practitioner became more apparent. However, becoming a nurse manager necessitated the inclusion of a foundation of traditional management theory in addition to my explorations into helicy and pandimensionality.

Soon I was reading about turn of the century experiments with 40-watt light bulbs in shoe factories and time/motion studies involving the number of bed baths that could be done in 45 minutes. Theories were presented that purport that there are basically two types of people in the working world: "lazy" and "not lazy." It was difficult for me to imagine how these theories had any constructive relevance to the science and art of nursing. Was it reasonable to suggest that the nursing profession embrace the same managerial principles and work ethics as corporate America, or were nurses justly accountable to their own codes of professional behavior and standards of work performance? How could a Theory X, Y, or Z, derived from studies on machinery foremen, apply to me as I was doing crisis intervention with a suicidal adolescent or helping another nurse through the same process? How could we adopt a managerial approach from an industrial psychologist who never had the experience of changing dirty linen from under a 300-pound comatose patient or of working the night shift on Christmas? Furthermore, I wondered if it were even necessary to look beyond our own, unique theoretical knowledge base to create a method of managing ourselves.

Rogers (1990) in addressing the unique nature of nursing asserted that it is "not a summation of principles and theories from other fields dealing with different phenomena and rooted in different paradigms" (p. 6). Rather, its uniqueness emanates from its concern with people and their environment, the purpose being to "promote health and well being for all persons wherever they are" (Rogers, 1992, p. 28). Given this, it would seem logical that a nurse manager would seek to engender this process, but that in addition to clients, nurses, and their work environments would be the focus of concern and caring.

Granted, this notion flew in the face of traditional management formulas, most of which seemed to be sequential improvements on how to get more workers to do more tasks, more expediently, with less money. Nevertheless, I felt that as a Rogerian nurse, I needed to assume a more humanistic approach in working with people. Serendipitously, a casual gesture during an informal meeting with one of my former professors, Pat Moccia, affirmed the belief in my convictions, and shaped the direction of my future explorations in nursing administration.

Pat was dean of a Nursing School at a major New York College, and as a mentor of mine, I called her for some career advice. Pat had invited me to campus for a cup of coffee to talk, and on the way to the cafeteria, she casually stopped by two of the department secretaries to ask if she could bring anything back for them. They smiled appreciatively, chatted a little, and gave Pat their order. She carefully wrote down each order and we proceeded to buy coffee and food for ourselves and the secretaries.

I was astonished! Pat was taking food orders for her secretaries! Moreover, it seemed as though this was a commonplace event. Wasn't it supposed to be the other way around? Weren't the department secretaries supposed to be asking THE DEAN what she wanted from the cafeteria?

I have always remembered that episode, for it occurred to me that the simple act of merely asking a coworker if they would like a cup of coffee is in and of itself, a pattern manifestation that expresses caring and concern. During the relative moment in time, the mutual process between Pat and the secretaries might be viewed as being "informal;" fluid, flowing, and easy-going (Butcher, 1994, p. 416). Informality characterized the mutually respectful, flexible, yet efficient way in which they worked together. It didn't matter that the departmental secretaries were technically "subordinate" to Pat in the organization. It didn't matter that traditional delegative logic was tossed aside. What *did* matter was that the artificial, arbitrary boundaries of the workplace were abandoned, giving rise to what might be considered pandimensional awareness.

Pandimensionality encompasses multiple realities (Butcher, 1994) and the uniqueness of individual human field patterns. An appreciation of pandimensionality provides us with a realistic perspective of ourselves in relation to other human and environmental fields. Pandimensionality helps us to understand that our lives and careers are not only in perpetual flux and unpredictable, but that they assume significance in accordance with the nature of our pattern manifestations and our mutual process with other human beings. Working in mutual process, human beings have the opportunity to experience heightened levels of cooperation and job satisfaction on the job when their focus of concern shifts away from the spatial or temporal limitations.

Pandimensionality invites us to approach workplace issues without the usual lines of demarcation between roles, titles, or tasks. Instead, we are valued for our own unique contributions to the wellness of human beings through our work. This may be accomplished through appraisal and consideration of the relative past, present, and future of our coworkers in the creation of a healthier work environment.

As Phillips noted (1994), the Science of Unitary Human Beings allows us to relinquish the need to control or dominate, and instead, focus on the potentiation of individuality. The creative use of power is one way in which the pandimensional nurse manager can motivate, inspire, and guide coworkers. The use of power in the Rogerian perspective is seen as a shared activity based on knowledge (Barrett, 1986), rather than a managerial tool of coercion or attempted manipulation. For example, should a staff member enjoy working with depressed clients, it would make sense to provide special opportunities for that individual to work with depressed clients even in a "medical-surgical" setting. If one displayed a continuing interest in this area, it would be advantageous to facilitate further explorations into learning about these opportunities. Cultivation of the unique talents and diverse interests of coworkers helps to foster a more evolved and healthier work environment, a process of change consistent with the Principles of Resonancy and Helicy.

The evaporation of perceived spatial and temporal boundaries may be a scary notion for the fledgling pandimensional nurse manager. For example, one potential dilemma of many nurse managers is whether or not to take an active part in the care of clients. Many nurses who cross the imaginary line into the dimension of management often act as though their purview no longer includes immediate, tactile client contact. The pandimensional nurse manager appreciates the opportunities to access multiple modes of awareness in practice through the process of integrality. Though it may not be necessary for a nurse manager to assume a client caseload every day, it is fortuitous to experience a wide panorama of workplace events, including the more direct aspects of client care.

However, being in a more pivotal position to facilitate workplace-environmental patterning, the pandimensional nurse manager might be concerned with questions such as "What does it 'feel' like to work here?" "How could we enhance (any number of things) in our work arena?" "What are the emerging needs of the people that we are in process with?" "What kind of work atmosphere do I want to try to create here?" The answers to these questions require the activation of objective and subjective appraisals, from wiping a client's brow to envisioning the right color scheme for a family conference room. Deliberate involvement in day-to-day operations also helps to generate more harmony among coworkers.

In addressing the use of metaphor in nursing, Smith (1992) writes "metaphors not only communicate meaning; they also suggest paths for action or practice" (p. 48). As Rogers (1970) described the practice of nursing as "promoting symphonic interaction" of human and environmental fields (p. 122), the pandimensional nurse manager is aware of the importance of promoting symphonic integrality with nurses and their environments. The metaphor of music making is particularly applicable to nursing and nursing management.

In many ways, being a nurse manager is like conducting an orchestra. A conductor must be aware of all the parts; the melodies in the string section, syncopation played by the brass section, and so on, but make them sound as one. He or she should be able to give a clear indication of where one is in the score at all times, while simultaneously conveying the feeling, intensity, and dynamics that the composer intended. Similarly, the nurse manager strives for clarity and direction without sacrificing sensitivity or feeling.

It is critical to understand, however, that despite the emotive dramatics that we enjoy watching while a conductor leads an orchestra, the *musicians* are primarily interested in knowing where they are in the score, the tempo the conductor wants and the precise beat and relative musical dynamics in the measure they're playing. In essence, the primary responsibility of being a conductor is to provide the members of the orchestra with a continuous metrical roadmap of sound through time in the shaping of an event that seems *timeless*. The technical considerations of the music making are already in place; musicians know their instruments, and are able to bring individuality and expressiveness to each piece, even while playing with others. All they need are musical guideposts along the way. Metaphorically speaking, the nurse manager who chooses to practice within the framework of the Science of Unitary Human Beings understands the paradoxical considerations of patterning an environmental field by providing what the staff needs in the fulfillment of their chosen work.

Congruently, one needs to resist the use of reductionistic approaches to problems and challenges. As James Levine, Artistic Director of the Metropolitan Opera notes (Chesterman, 1992), nowhere in history are there references to composers complaining about a "sour" note by a horn or string player in a performance of their work. Rather, their criticisms indicate that a performance failed to "capture the right spirit, the right character, the right motivation" (Chesterman, 1992, p. 153) that the work was intended to convey. Nurse managers who focus on "sour notes" (e.g., "poor performances," or mistakes) and spend all day writing up disciplinary notes on employees may be ignoring the "big" picture; that is, the spirit, the nature, and the mission of their work.

The pandimensional nurse manager, not unlike a conductor interpreting a Brahms symphony, a composer, or a sculptor, is visionary in conceptualizing the creation of a new form of expression that reflects his or her individuality. For some nurses, it may be the development of a support group for Alzheimer's caregivers, or collaboration with other nurses interested in starting a consulting firm. Others may choose to write articles or books, or chronicle their perceptions of life through the lens of a 35 mm camera.

A personal, recurring vision of mine is to imagine the creation of a "Health Patterning Tune-Up Shop," styled after "Astor Place Haircutters" in New York City, a two-story, no-frills, high-volume barber shop that boasts dozens of highly efficient hair stylists who give precise, individualized haircuts at a fraction of the price one would pay in a salon. However, instead of haircuts, the "Tune-Up Shop" would be staffed with an

array of owner-manager nurses, who for a reasonable fee, would be able
to provide Therapeutic Touch sessions, consultations on career counseling, stress reduction, or human field mutual process disturbances, educa-
tive sessions on specific health concerns, or other health patterning
modalities without expense or delay. The term "tune-up" is chosen to
convey the concept of healing, the enhancement of life, and gentle crafts-
manship, as well as a sense of harmonic and rhythmic well-being. Not unlike a concert hall filled with the sounds of a cacophonous orchestra
oscillating toward tonal synchrony in the moments before the down-beat
of a conductor, the "Tune-Up Shop" would be bristling with anticipation
and excitement as human potentials become actualized, power profiles
enhanced, and pattern manifestations heightened. Unlimited opportunities exist for the nurse who is willing to abandon an allegiance to traditional, predetermined nursing roles. Yet, the evolution of our procreative
efforts is integral with our attitudes about the way in which we choose to
work with people.

On a cold Saturday morning in December 1984, I began my first day as
a nurse manager in a 45-bed, acute-care psychiatric floor. I knew none of
the staff or cliients. I walked onto the unit gingerly, half-smiling, and said,
"Hi—I'm Bela . . . the new weekend nursing supervisor. How's it going?"
"Lousy," replied a nameless face. "We're out of coffee! Someone forgot to
buy a new can." Remembering that morning with Pat, I knew just what to
do. "No problem," I replied. "Tell me what you want—I'll go to the donut
shop on the corner."

The staff looked at me as though I was a bit peculiar, but it didn't
seem to matter. They needed their morning coffee. As for me, the opportunity to provide it for them was the beginning of what was to become a tremendously gratifying, mutually rewarding working process
that lasted for years.

As a Rogerian nurse manager, I have come to believe the following:
Human beings like being acknowledged for their talents and appreciated
for their uniqueness; life is becoming more complicated and unpredictable, both personally and professionally; and, deliberative patterning
can be quite a risky endeavor for a nursing administrator. But as Rogers
(1990) said, "enjoy your forays into the unknown" (p. 11). Being a nurse
manager is a three-dimensional ticket to a pandimensional trip.

REFERENCES

Barrett, E. A. M. (1986). Investigation of the principle of helicy: The relationship
    of human field motion and power. In V. Malinski (Ed.), *Explorations on*

Martha Rogers' science of unitary human beings (pp. 173-184). Norwalk, CT: Appleton-Century-Crofts.

Butcher, H. K. (1994). The Unitary Field Pattern Portrait method: Development of a research method for Rogers' science of unitary human beings. In M. Madrid & E. A. M. Barrett (Eds.), *Rogers' scientific art of nursing practice* (pp. 397-429). New York: NLN Press.

Chesterman, R. (1992). *Conductors in conversation.* London: Robson.

Phillips, J. R. (1994). The open-ended nature of the science of unitary beings. In M. Madrid & E. A. M. Barrett (Eds.), *Rogers' scientific art of nursing practice* (pp. 11-25). New York: NLN Press.

Rogers, M. E. (1970). *An introduction to the theoretical bases of nursing.* Philadelphia: Davis.

Rogers, M. E. (1990). Nursing: Science of unitary, irreducible, human beings: Updated 1990. In E. A. M. Barrett (Ed.), *Visions of Rogers' science-based nursing* (pp. 5-11). New York: NLN Press.

Rogers, M. E. (1992). Nursing science and the space age. *Nursing Science Quarterly, 5,* 27-34.

Smith, M. C. (1992). Metaphor in nursing theory. *Nursing Science Quarterly, 5*(2), 48-49.

19

Therapeutic Touch: A Model for Community-Based Health Promotion

Katherine E. Matas

*T*he Therapeutic Touch and Centering Clinic at Arizona State University (ASU) College of Nursing opened in May of 1992 after one year of developmental work. A proposal, submitted to the academic administration of the College, was approved and much was learned from meeting with the director of ASU's nurse-managed Community Services Clinic and collegial consultations at the Center for Human Caring, University of Colorado in Denver.

The setting for the clinic is a bright and cheerful room in the College of Nursing. There is carpeting on the floor and a large window that overlooks the campus's trees and flowers. Initial advertising was an announcement placed in the College of Nursing faculty mailboxes and student dockets. The volume of interested persons was remarkable. Within several weeks of operation, new participants had to wait three weeks for an appointment, and as of June 1996, this pattern has not changed.

The clinic, open only one day a week, was established as a pilot research project. The broad purpose was health promotion with a focus on outcome measurement. The clinic flyer stated "Therapeutic Touch is an approach to healing derived from the laying on of hands. It is a holistic modality for actualizing innate healing capacities. Centering is a self power-enhancing skill that can be learned to assist in moving more smoothly through changes related to health and well being." The target population has been the ASU faculty, staff, and students. There has been no charge for services, as this was a pilot research project. All individuals sign a consent to participate and are free to discontinue involvement at any time.

THE CLINIC EXPERIENCE

Since 1992, a total of 65 people have participated in the Therapeutic Touch (Krieger, 1979, 1993) and Centering Clinic. The primary source of referral is word of mouth, that is, hearing about the clinic from another participant or curiosity about Therapeutic Touch. The University's Employee Assistance Program has also made referrals to the clinic.

Presenting health situations are diverse. At the first clinic appointment, each participant is asked to identify a health potential to be working toward. Data collection consists of translating the goal into a Visual Analogue Scale (VAS) (Gift, 1989) and obtaining the history using a form that records demographic information, general health history, and current health practices. Open-ended questions on the history form include:

What do you consider your special talents and interests?

Why have you come to the clinic at this time?

Is there anything else you would like and/or need to tell me at this time?

Clinic appointments average one hour in length. Most participants have 2 to 5 appointments. Skills for self healing are taught to direct people toward greater well-being. Teaching is begun at the first visit and continued through subsequent visits. It is explained to all clients that personal commitment and active participation are necessary in order to work in a mutual process of change. Therapeutic Touch and centering are explained and background information is shared. Information is also shared on the Science of Unitary Human Beings (Rogers, 1986, 1990) and Barrett's power theory (Barrett, 1990). Handouts are given on Therapeutic Touch and centering exercises. Participants are asked to practice centering daily and are given a log to record their experiences (Figure 19.1). Specific centering images, based on the information accessed during the Therapeutic Touch experience, are suggested.

Additional reading or exercises may be suggested at the first visit, depending on the initial presenting health situation. This, however, is more commonly suggested at subsequent visits. Referrals given to participants may range from counseling to alternative health practitioners to allopathic physicians.

The first and second appointments lie from one week to one month apart. Factors that determine when the participant will return include the nature of the presenting situation, availability of appointments, and participant schedules.

At the beginning of the second visit and at each subsequent visit, the participant is asked to complete a Visual Analogue Scale (VAS) for their identified goals (Gift, 1989). Discussion then focuses on progress or difficulties in their "well being work." Their centering experience is explored with the use of the completed centering log. Modifications in centering practice are discussed, for example, changing the visual image they used, focusing on their breath, or centering during an activity. Mindfulness meditations of Tich Nhat Hahn (1976) or Kabat-Zinn (1990) may also be introduced at this time as an aid to centering. Concepts and principles from the Science of Unitary Human Beings and Barrett's power theory are discussed and explored at each visit: How do they knowingly participate in change? What is their experience of integrality like?

"Homework" from the second visit includes continued practice with centering and individualized readings, including stories, novels, poetry, and self-help books that may inform each individual. Completion of the Life Grid (Figure 19.2) may also be suggested. The Life Grid is a modification of the Peak Performances Grid (Garfield, 1984). At the second or third visit, many participants are ready to look at their well-being in the context of the global picture of their life. The completed Life Grid (Figure 19.2) serves as an inventory of activities, attitudes, life events, and so on, that individuals consider helpful or harmful to themselves, and serves as introductory work to exploration of life process and purpose (Appendix 19.A; Spencer & Adams, 1990).

Therapeutic Touch takes place 30–40 minutes after the appointment begins and lasts 10–20 minutes. A brief discussion of the Therapeutic Touch experience concludes the visit. All participants take 10–15 minutes after the appointment to sit quietly so that they can obtain full benefit from the relaxation response and energy work.

From the practitioner's standpoint, a major aspect of practice in working with people over time is the process that unfolds naturally. However,

Figure 19.1   Daily Centering Log

Today's Date: _____

Frequency of Centering

Morning _____

Afternoon _____

Evening _____

Night _____

Ease of Centering

Morning _____

Afternoon _____

Evening _____

Night _____

Quality of Centering
(Description of experience: For example, What? How? Where? When? Why?)

Copyright © K. Matas 1992.

Figure 19.2   Life Grid

Fill in activities in the appropriate grid below:

Top Left: Things you want to do, but are not doing.
Top Right: Things you want to do and are doing.
Bottom Right: Things you are doing but do not want to do.
Bottom Left: Things you are not doing and do not want to do.

	Things You Are Not Doing.	Things You Are Doing.
Things You Want to Do.		
Things You Do Not Want to Do.		

Adapted from Garfield (1984).

there is a guiding framework which is not rigidly adhered to during the sessions. The framework has two major components:

Laboratory of the Self: Part One

- Discovering oneself and environment as energy fields in mutual process.
- Experience and application in daily life.
- Therapeutic touch.
- Centering.
- Exercises/energy work.

Laboratory of the Self: Part Two

- Who/what am I in process with in my environment?
- Who/what is most significant to me in the mutual processing of my human/environmental field?
- Life purpose work.
- Therapeutic touch.
- Centering.
- Exercises.

The outcome data for the clinic's pilot project were measured by the Visual Analogue Scale (VAS). Participants identified the health potential they considered most important to be working toward. Each end of the VAS was used as a bipolar representation of how close they were to achieving their ideal. They chose the words, placed at the appropriate end, that best described how far away or near they were toward reaching their goals. From this description, it can be seen that the VAS was used (in this study) in a similar manner to the use of the semantic differential (Osgood, Succi, & Tannenbaum, 1957) or the Cantrill Ladder (McKeehan, Cowling, & Wykle, 1986). The purpose of this method is to have participants sense or feel their change process in relation to their goal (Figure 19.3).

A central objective of the Therapeutic Touch and Centering Clinic is to test a model of practice that includes data collection for outcome measurement. This method of developing data collection would not be intrusive but integral to the clinical process and, more ideally, would be valued by participants. It could, therefore, be easily incorporated into the therapeutic mutual process.

Record forms were developed that included the initial history form, a narrative record sheet with human body figures to record Therapeutic Touch findings, and blank VAS forms. Each VAS and narrative form has

Figure 19.3   Visual Analogue Scale Examples

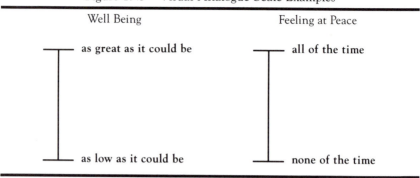

the visit number recorded on it. Narrative notes include a summary of participant progress and self-insights. Discussion topics, teaching information, summary impressions and next phase of the mutual process plan are also recorded. This method of charting is similar to the Subjective, Objective, Assessment, Plan format (SOAP), recognizing that each category reflects a perspective occurring in mutual process. A more accurate acronym for this documentation process would be MAP (mutual process, attunement, plan).

Body Figures (Figure 19.4) are used to document Therapeutic Touch. If additional space is needed, the narrative area is used. A numerical scale ranging from 0 to 4 is used to indicate strength of the field. Zero indicates void areas, 4 indicates excessive flow, 2 indicates an open "normal" flow. Use of the numbers 1 and 3 indicate a relative deficit or excess patterning process of the field. Symbols are frequently drawn on or around the body figure to indicate more qualitative findings and impressions. For example, a jagged line may be drawn over the head and shoulders to indicate a rough, disturbed quality of the field. Short notes of particular images or impressions that were part of the Therapeutic Touch experience may also be recorded near the body figure.

Preliminary Client Outcomes

Data analysis has been completed for the first 53 participants. Ninety percent report improvement or progress toward their goal. These data are based on the initial VAS, before the first Therapeutic Touch experience and the VAS recorded at the last visit. The mean magnitude of change toward identified goals was 42 percent.

Figure 19.4   Body Figures

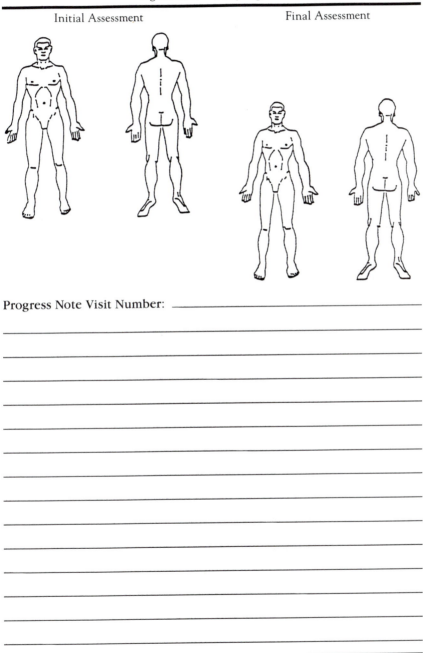

Initial Assessment   Final Assessment

Progress Note Visit Number: _____

_____

_____

_____

_____

_____

_____

_____

_____

_____

_____

_____

_____

_____

_____

_____

_____

CONCLUSION

This pilot research project will serve as a foundation for the continuing development of a scientist-practitioner (Barlow, Hayes, & Nelson, 1985) and an evolving, organic model (Chenault, 1975) of Rogerian nursing practice. In this practice model, Therapeutic Touch serves multiple functions for participants that includes a lived experience of pandimensional mutual field process and an intentional act of health promotion. The person's active participation and commitment to personal well-being are also essential in this model of practice.

The Therapeutic Touch and Centering Clinic was renamed the Health Patterning Clinic in July of 1995 when it became a formal component of the ASU Employee Wellness Program. The use of Rogerian nursing modalities, such as those utilized in this practice model, can be easily integrated into community-based healthcare and are particularly appropriate for health promotion and wellness, and partnering with other services such as Employee Assistance Programs (EAPs), case management, and school health (Matas, 1996).

Data collection methods, particularly those in relation to personal centering practice and experiences with self-healing strategies, will be refined in the next phase of developing the model. Ideally, this practice model will be tested by other practitioners. The potential benefit of incorporating outcome measurement as an integral part of science-based practice is unlimited and has implications for data-based healthcare reform at the forefront.

APPENDIX 19.A*

Life Purpose

Sages throughout the ages have observed the importance of examining one's life. The questions "Who am I?" and "Why am I here?" are not meant to be rhetorical, although the answers are elusive and can seem impossible to answer at times. BUT, finding the answers are worth the effort because clarity, strength, peace and well-being may result.

Clues to your life purpose abound in daily life if you know what to look for. For example, what in your life gives you a deep sense of satisfaction, of completion, of happiness? What are those things that "make your heart

---

*Copyright K. Matas 1992.

sing"? Consider the times you have felt like this. What were you doing at the time? What were you thinking and feeling? Were you alone or with others? Probe until you have distilled the essence of those things that make you feel fulfilled. A cross-check for the accuracy of your conclusions is how you feel at the end of the process. If you have accurately discerned, there will be a resonance that occurs within you—a feeling of deep knowing, and a sense of being energized, vibrant.

There are also techniques or methods that can facilitate the examination process described above. Generally, an activity that lifts you above or beyond the hassles of daily life will be helpful. Listening to an inspirational piece of music or going for a walk in a beautiful natural setting are examples of such activities. Contemplation is another activity very helpful to this process. Many methods of contemplation exist. Choose one comfortable or familiar to you. Examples include prayer, meditation, and centering. Prerequisite to effective contemplation is physical and mental relaxation. Without this, our body/mind is still in a whir, which prevents reaching the gentle, calm state necessary for contemplation.

Above all, don't push too hard or rush yourself. The process of determining your life purpose is one that naturally unfolds. Each individual walks a unique path. You will not know what lies beyond a door until you open it and walk through.

Listen to the cues your own life has provided for you. Take note and then probe those events and times which brought deep happiness and satisfaction to you. You will find many doors to open which may lead to the untold treasures of the unique beauty of who and what you are, as well as why you are here.

Life Purpose Exercise

Go for a walk alone in a peaceful place or put on your favorite inspirational music at a time when there will be no interruptions. Have a paper and pencil handy.

Consciously LET GO of the usual "chatter" that fills your mind. Let the tension you are holding in your body flow out with each breath you exhale. Become centered.

As you enter this experience, all the while feeling more deeply relaxed and "empty" of your daily concerns, begin to remember the times you have felt exceptionally well. You will know those times by the vibrant sense of well-being you felt, the elation, the exuberance, the connectedness.

If no time like this comes to mind, don't panic. Go more deeply into the music or look for the natural beauty surrounding you as you walk. Continue to LET GO any remaining tension—when you are more deeply relaxed and detached from daily pressure, you will remember (a) happy time(s).

When you are in touch with the happy experience, examine it closely. Select one if several come to mind. Observe yourself from as many angles as possible. Ask questions like: What? When? How? Where? Why? Stretch and expand yourself as much as possible to see that part of you that was affirmed and honored in the experience.

When you have observed all that there is to "see," take out the paper and pencil and describe the event. Can you draw any conclusions about yourself? What have you discovered or remembered about yourself? Perhaps drawing a picture can more accurately capture your expression than words.

Describe the following

The event or occasion: _____

_____

The environment or conditions surrounding this time: _____

_____

My special quality that was active at this time: _____

_____

Do I currently have opportunity to use this special quality? _____

_____

A drawing representative (symbolic or otherwise) of this special quality:

_____

_____

REFERENCES

Barlow, D. H., Hayes, S. C., & Nelson, R. O. (1985). *The scientist practitioner: Research and accountability in clinical and educational settings.* Elmsford, NY: Pergamon Press.

Barrett, E. A. M. (1990). Health patterning with clients in a private environment. In E. A. M. Barrett (Ed.), *Visions of Rogers' science-based nursing* (pp. 105–115). New York: NLN Press.

Chenault, J. (1975). *Human services educational and practice: An organic model.* New York: Behavioral Publications.

Garfield, C. (1984). *Peak performance.* Los Angeles: Warner Books.

Gift, A. G. (1989). Visual analogue scales: Measurement of subjective phenomena. *Nursing Research, 38*(5), 286–288.

Kabat-Zinn, J. (1990). *Full catastrophe living: Using the wisdom of your body and mind to face stress, pain, and illness.* New York: Delacorte Press.

Krieger, D. (1979). *The therapeutic touch: How to use your hands to help or to heal.* Englewood Cliffs, NJ: Prentice-Hall.

Krieger, D. (1993). *Accepting your power to heal: The personal practice of therapeutic touch.* Santa Fe, NM: Bear & Company.

Matas, K. E. (1996). Continuity of care and community based nursing. In R. Craven & C. Hinkle (Eds.). *Fundamentals of nursing* (pp. 108–121). Philadelphia: J. B. Lippincott.

McKeehan, K. M., Cowling, W. R., & Wykle, M. L. (1986). Central self anchoring ladders: Methodological considerations for nursing science. In P. L. Chinn (Ed.), *Nursing research methodology* (pp. 285–294). Rockville, MD: Aspen.

Nhat Hahn, T. (1976). *The miracle of mindfulness.* Boston: Beacon Press.

Osgood, C. E., Succi, G. J., & Tannenbaum, P. H. (1957). *The measurement of meaning.* Chicago: University of Illinois Press.

Rogers, M. E. (1986). Science of unitary human beings. In V. M. Malinski (Ed.), *Explorations on Martha Rogers' science of unitary human beings* (pp. 3–8). Norwalk, CT: Appleton-Century-Crofts.

Rogers, M. E. (1990). Nursing: Science of unitary, irreducible human beings: Update 1990. In E. A. M. Barrett (Ed.), *Visions of Rogers' science-based nursing* (pp. 5–11). New York: NLN Press.

Spencer, S. A., & Adams, J. D. (1990). *Life changes: Growing through personal transitions.* San Louis Obispo, CA: Impact.

20

A Celebration of Unitary Human Beings: Becoming a Mother

Diane Poulios

*B*ecoming a mother is a whole new world of challenges and discoveries, growth and change, wholeness and unity. My belly was swelling, my stomach was retching; my hands were shaky; and my eyes were red. My emotions were dramatic and my visions were startling. They told me I was pregnant! Who was I becoming?

I was emerging as a young girl, a daughter, and a granddaughter; a woman, a wife, and a mother; an older woman, a grandmother, and a great grandmother. Such becomingness makes sense within a pandimensional framework of unfolding patterns in human time.

Stories are "an expression of human consciousness and a means to expand and move toward wholeness" (Sandelowski, 1994, p. 30). This is a story of early motherhood colored in Rogerian shades of bright bold colors and pastel hues; a kaleidoscope of experiences, thoughts, and visions of a maternal world.

Becoming a mother: what does it mean? It means wholeness and change. Bohm's theory of implicate order suggests the presence of a universal wholeness that transcends all life (Malinski, 1990). As I look inward, I can follow the underground stream that unites all maternal awareness. Lemkow (1991) states that wholeness encourages the wisdom of cooperation, tolerance, sharing, love, and compassion. Aren't these expressions of motherhood? Wholeness embraces the dynamic patterns manifested of the mother-child group field. Both change, yet remain as one throughout life.

The Rogerian Theory of Unitary Human Beings has facilitated my understanding of motherhood. It has been a magic carpet enabling me to journey through new dimensions and understand the process at each helical turn. Rogers (1992) identifies human beings and their respective environments as energy fields. An energy field is a unifying concept expressing wholeness and dynamism. Change highlights Rogers' (1992) principles of homeodynamics. All human and environmental fields manifest wave patterns of varying frequencies. Rogers perceives life as an open system of creative and accelerating wave patterns increasing in diversity and occurring within a pandimensional framework without spatial or temporal boundaries.

Openness, pattern, pandimensionality, and human time are matrices of the human field image. Phillips (1990) defines the human field image as an evolving diverse manifestation of the human field pattern. It emerges out of the synthesis of past, present, and future experiences, creating a pandimensional image of the human being. According to Rogers, time is experienced as a whole in the relative present (Malinski, 1990). Paletta (1990) identifies human time as a temporal experience allowing measurement in relation to human patterns incorporating increased diversity, innovation, creativity, and imagination. The human field image is an irreducible whole that provides definition to one's becoming within a human time framework.

Pregnancy and childbirth are best described as human field image experiences. The growing fetus is a human energy field embraced within another. Pregnancy is a pandimensional extension of the manifestation of the mother's human field image in continuous process with her environmental field. The infant field unfolds out of the maternal field with its own separate and unique environmental field. The human field images of mother and unborn child are separate yet whole, each manifesting its own diverse energy pattern, yet creatively becoming as one. In *To be a woman,* Speeth (1990) writes,

> *Gracefully do the mother and child give attention and gratefully receive it, as with one mind. In the beginning baby and mother are one, and that one is baby. Thus the divinity the mother sees in her newborn is also hers. (p. 114)*

Is this motherhood? To experience my own unfolding through the emerging field of an unborn child?

The mutual processing of baby and mother's unfolding human field patterns manifested unexpectedly. My husband and I said goodbye prior to vacationing in Mexico with my parents. I needed a respite and he was unable to accompany me. On the plane, I thought about the years we had attempted to conceive; all the procedures, medications, and pain we had experienced. My human field image felt numb. However, the closer I flew toward Cancun, the more I could sense my energy rhythms. I began to feel more aware of my integrality with the universe.

Ironically, instead of feeling rested in Cancun, I felt as if I was buzzing with a strange energy frequency; I was unable to sleep. Each night I awoke abruptly, as if disturbed by diverse energy forms in the room. Was I resonating with and becoming unusually sensitive to the subtle energy field vibrations manifesting from fecund spirits of ancient Mayan civilizations in pandimensional time? I looked out at the ocean and heard the rhythmic sounds of the water. I did not know I was already pregnant; I would discover this upon my return home.

As human time unfolded, the growing fetus declared its becomingness with great strength and intensity. My human field patterns were spiraling at such a frequency that I developed hyperemesis gravidarum. I felt overwhelmed, excited, and afraid of losing what I wanted so much; but I sensed my child's will to live. I visualized its heartbeat on the ultrasound screen. It was like a flickering star determined to sparkle through any environmental field. The small energy field within me communicated its message: "I am here, so pay attention!" I felt somewhat intimidated by this powerful energy field that I perceived as taking control of my body.

Through prayer and meditation, I encouraged the resonancy of our fields toward greater harmony. I visualized soothing blue colors and listened to soft music. I experienced an awareness of the symbol of Mother Mary and her powers of nurturance, wholeness, and compassion. Through her wisdom, I participated knowingly in the patterning of our integral energy fields (Barrett, 1986). Self-administered Therapeutic Touch was attempted, but the sensation felt too stimulating on my changing human field. The gentle patterning of imagery was a peaceful therapy for my discomfort. The high frequency of smell created havoc in my stomach. I strived to create a scent-free environment, which was a challenge, providing my scent-full environmental field.

As field patterns of mother and baby emerged, manifesting greater harmony and higher frequency, the perceived sense of chaos seemed to wane. I was finally able to eat, take vitamins, and drink fluids. A new strength slowly emerged within me.

I enjoyed my changing human field through the rhythmic movements of swimming. The blueness of the water and its sensual flow over my skin calmed my anxieties. I sensed waves of peace and tranquility. Time seemed to stop as I experienced a oneness with my baby and the rhythm of life. I felt weightless and expansive underwater, and it seemed as if my human field was everywhere, resonating in a frequency I had never experienced before. Fear of this dynamic process transformed into awe.

Pregnancy changes more than one's body image. The size of my growing abdomen seemed to accurately reflect my feelings of transcending perceived human field boundaries. In addition, my human field patterns manifested more assertive, expressive, and open behaviors.

Within the human time of 16 weeks, fetal movement began. There was no fluttering, just a big kick in the side. The fetal energy field was communicating its human field image. It was a boy—intense, strong, and quite spirited. My husband and I laughed at the display of such toughness from a little being. We named him Nicholas.

I attempted Therapeutic Touch again. Upon appraisal, I sensed the high-frequency pattern of his energy field and was aware that he was receptive to relaxation and centering. I focused on wholeness and compassion throughout the treatment and sensed his relaxed state. His frequent movements stopped and he started moving again when I completed the process. My field seemed to resonate with the high-frequency patterning that manifested during Therapeutic Touch, whether I was treating other people or concentrating on him. This phenomenon seemed to intensify my capacity as a caregiver. Our unique oneness created a powerful medium for the mutual process of healing.

Colors transmit varying frequencies of energy wave patterns (von Rohr, 1992). They are powerful reflectors of the human field image. My energy field frequency resonated with the vibrations from the color green. According to von Rohr, green symbolizes calm, growth, and new life. The baby's room was painted light green with water colors in the crib. There was a flowlike quality to the colors, reflecting the swimming rhythmic patterns we had experienced.

I grew big and tired. I experienced time as creeping and felt I would be pregnant forever. The mutual processing of our changing field rhythms manifested in severe Braxton-Hicks contractions. I had to stop working and rest. I took slow walks to continue my exercise and emerge with another unfolding energy wave spiral.

On a beautiful fall day in October, I walked amidst the colorful foliage. I harmonized with nature's rhythms of wholeness and change. In an instant of timelessness, a black cat with deep black eyes patterned its step alongside mine. The cat looked straight into my eyes and silently said,

"Your baby is coming now," then ran away. The pandimensional quality of the experience shook me. I returned home in disbelief, with its eyes engraved on my mind. A few hours later I went into labor.

Waves of vise-like pain enveloped my abdomen occurring in a rhythmic tempo, crescendoing as the time grew near to depart for the hospital. Lamaze breathing exercises helped me to resonate with accelerating energy field rhythms. Already sleep-deprived from physical discomfort, I entered the human timeframe of continued wakefulness. My husband and I drove to the hospital at twilight, feeling excited, nervous, and elated.

The waves of uterine movement unfolded increasingly. At 1:00 PM, Nicholas began to crown. With my husband's support, and the guidance of my nurse and obstetrician, strength emerged from the depths of my being. I felt that I was no longer of this world and had no physical body. I was beyond pain and exhaustion. My human field image was transcending to give birth to another human being of greater diversity and higher frequency than my husband or me. Along with my newborn, I felt that I, too, was born! As Nicholas lay on my stomach looking into my eyes, I experienced only him and my husband. We were as one in a pandimensional world of ecstasy! Time and the tears of joy were continuous and unbroken.

Baby Nicholas was a challenge! A mother's worst nightmare—a colicky baby—he cried incessantly from his second day of birth. Frantically, my husband and I offered him everything we knew. He curled his feet up under his belly and wailed in pain after each feeding. There was no such thing as bedtime. I attempted Therapeutic Touch, wondering if he would recognize the patterning process he experienced in the womb. No luck. However, the appraisal did confirm my awareness of chaotic energy and what felt like abdominal congestion.

The strong love I felt for my son was beyond expression. Nicholas' field pattern manifested a sense of discomfort for a new life. Night after night I walked him, crying tears he was physically unable to shed. I felt his pain and frustration with this new world.

I realized that Nicholas resonated and seemed to relax with the patterning processes of warmth, melody, a soft voice, and touch. I sensed he could understand me as I repeated, "Mommy's here. I know you're hurting." He quieted at the sound of my voice. Lullabies and classical music, integrated with motion, lulled him to sleep.

As Nicholas' becomingness unfolded through maturation and increasingly diverse energy field patterns, his discomfort subsided and he was able to reveal new dimensions. Nick mirrored the human field image he portrayed during my pregnancy, a sensitive boy with spirit, will, and great intensity of character. To this day, he stares up at me with his unusual deep black eyes as if heralding my innermost thoughts. At that relative present, that pandimensional black cat emerges within those very eyes.

My Rogerian world of motherhood has allowed me to profoundly experience the wholeness and rich changes in life. Through a new perception of humanness, I perceive every child as my child and feel at one with the universe. I am inspired by the courage and strength of women, and hold deep reverence for the special pandimensional mother-child group field bond. As a former nun exclaimed:

> *The whole universe is a miracle. The idea of an infant developing in you being a special mystery . . . well, that's no more wonderful than it would be developing in somebody else, some other woman, or the little kitten in the mamma cat. Why can't we become ecstatic over developing life, period? We're constantly participating in it whether we're pregnant or not!"*
> *(Anderson & Hopkins, 1991, p. 78)*

REFERENCES

Anderson, S. R., & Hopkins, P. (1991). *The feminine face of God.* New York: Bantam Books.

Barrett, E. A. M. (1986). Investigation of the principle of helicy: The relationship of human field motion and power. In V. M. Malinski (Ed.), *Explorations on Martha Rogers' science of unitary human beings* (pp. 173-184). Norwalk, CT: Appleton-Century-Crofts.

Lemkow, K. A. (1991, December). *A note on evolution: The wholeness principle.* New York: New York Theosophical Society.

Malinski, V. M. (1990). The meaning of a progressive world view in nursing. In M. L. Chaska (Ed.), *The nursing profession: Turning points* (pp. 237-244). St. Louis: Mosby.

Paletta, J. L. (1990). The relationship of temporal experience to human time. In E. A. M. Barrett (Ed.), *Visions of Rogers' science-based nursing* (pp. 239-253). New York: NLN Press.

Phillips, J. R. (1990). Changing human potentials and future visions of nursing: A human field image perspective. In E. A. M. Barrett (Ed.), *Visions of Rogers' science-based nursing* (pp. 13-25). New York: NLN Press.

Rogers, M. E. (1992). Nursing science and the space age. *Nursing Science Quarterly, 5*(1), 27-34.

Sandelowski, M. (1994). We are the stories we tell: Narrative knowing in nursing practice. *Journal of Holistic Nursing, 12*(1), 23-33.

Speeth, K. R. (1990). The Madonna. In C. Zweig (Ed.), *To be a woman.* Los Angeles: Jeremy A. Tarcher.

von Rohr, I. (1992). *Harmony is the healer.* Rockport, MA: Element.

21

A Plea to Educate
the Public About
Martha Rogers' Science of
Unitary Human Beings

Anita Mandl

I am not a nurse or health professional; I'm a businessperson who was exposed to Rogerian nursing while I was a patient at a major medical center.

I was scared.

I was uncomprehending and angry.

I was short-tempered toward a physician who, while probing my body, never addressed me or looked at me. He was talking to his residents about me while never acknowledging me.

In everyday life, I am an intelligent, professional, living a full life crammed with activities, family, and culture. Suddenly I seemed to become:

A victim.

A frightened and confused woman.

A patient who rationally understood what was happening during this pancreatitis attack, but also a woman who was emotionally distraught and felt out of control.

In 1989, I was a patient, unexpectedly, and like many people in this circumstance, trying desperately to reconcile my rational thinking about what was going on with my feeling of helplessness.

For me, the first day in the hospital emergency room, and then in a semi-private room, was bewildering and frightening. Nurses, doctors, aides were all talking around me, but rarely to me; tests were taken, blood was drawn, machines were hooked up, and I gathered that I'd need to stay for a few days to be monitored. Did I have a choice? Sure, I could just walk out, but I was feeling poorly and decided to stay.

At about 11:00 PM that night, a nurse came in to talk to me, explaining that she heard that I had an altercation with a physician and she asked if I wanted to talk about it. Did I imagine this? We talked, and talked, and talked. I heard stories; I told stories. We intermingled our tales and exchanged our experiences. I didn't realize just how angry and scared I was until we started talking. She massaged my body, held my hand, stroked my head, adjusted the pillows and the tubes, all the while soothing me with words and touch. I wasn't sure what was happening but what the hell, it felt great, so I let it happen. I was calmed, I felt understood, I received compassion and healing; my entire body and mind felt different, relaxed, and ready for whatever was to come next.

I didn't know it at the time, but this was my introduction to Rogerian nursing—what a gift.

As a result of my experience and my developing friendship with that nurse, Mary Madrid, I took an interest in learning about Martha Rogers. It's not easy for a layperson to "get into" Rogers. I found it difficult, but worth the struggle. I've done some wonderful work with a Rogerian health patterner (thank you, Elizabeth Barrett) and I've met many members of the Society of Rogerian Scholars. I've read (and understood some of) Martha's writing, which brings me to the point of this piece: Why can't Martha Rogers' philosophy and practice be known beyond the health profession?

Let's take Martha Rogers' thinking beyond the realm of healthcare practitioners and "mainstream" her. She is so "of today." Let's educate the general public, whether ill or well, about the possibilities of a change in healthcare by explaining Rogers' beliefs. Let those people who are hungry for alternative ways to look at health and illness know about the Science of Unitary Human Beings (SUHB). Let's watch as people discover their power to change their expectations about healthcare and let's help people find different ways to approach health issues for themselves and their loved ones.

Wouldn't it be great to see:

- Martha Rogers' face on tee-shirts all around the world.
- Schools, education facilities, and hospitals showing videos, giving patients and potential patients an understanding of health possibilities they may not have considered.
- Books, lectures, pamphlets, and dialogues explaining in layperson's terms, about the SUHB.
- A PBS series on the SUHB.
- Government funding, lobbying, conventions, and health conferences that include Martha Rogers' philosophies and possibilities for change in healthcare.
- Martha Rogers become a new Deepak Chopra, opening people's minds and thoughts to a deeper level.

I realize how difficult it is to translate Rogers' teachings into understandable language for the general public, but I believe it's worth the effort. Being ill might be a wake-up call for many of us to see the needed changes in healthcare as it did for me. All of us, not just nursing professionals, can help to break the paradigm, gain power, and transform our lives along with transforming healthcare practice and the healthcare expectations of millions of people.

22

Rogers in Reality: Staff Nurse Application of the Science of Unitary Human Beings in the Clinical Setting Following Changes in an Orientation Program

Tracey A. Woodward and Judy Heggie

*L*earning a nursing conceptual framework takes thought, effort, and time (Fitch et al., 1991). We had one hour, not a day, not a week, but sixty minutes to introduce new nursing employees to the conceptual framework of Martha Rogers' Science of Unitary Human Beings. This was the challenge presented to the Nursing Education Department of the San Diego Department of Veterans Affairs Medical Center (SDVAMC) in 1991, a challenge that initially seemed overwhelming. Some nursing leaders describe this model as abstract and difficult to implement, with individuals often struggling to understand the principles (Falco & Lobo, 1995). A reorganization took place in 1991 that would increase the scope of Nursing Service employees. The service would now include clerical staff, health technicians, as well as professional nurses who would need orientation, including an overview of healthcare as it relates to our facility.

HISTORY OF ROGERS' MODEL IMPLEMENTATION AT VAMC, SAN DIEGO

In 1984, a special projects committee within Nursing Service reviewed nursing theories and selected Rogers' conceptual framework for provision of nursing care (Heggie, Schoenmehl, Chang, & Grieco, 1989). Nursing Service acknowledged the benefit of establishing a common view of the client to guide practice, in part due to the unique nature of our federal hospital. San Diego county maintains two large military bases. As personnel relocate to our community, family members often seek employment with the VAMC, San Diego. VA regulations allow our facility to hire nurses with current licensure from any of the fifty states. The nurses employed here have varying educational backgrounds: approximately half have associate degrees, and many were educated in another country. While employment guidelines have enriched our department by bringing together healthcare personnel of diverse backgrounds, we noted that the view of health, human beings, nursing, and environment varied, based on that diversity. Implementation of Rogers' model encouraged a common view of our clients and their families as unitary, indivisible, irreducible human and environmental fields (Malinski, 1993).

The inservice provided during the first five years of implementation met with mixed reviews. In 1986, staff struggled to comprehend the significance of a purple slinky toy, used as a metaphor for helicy. Programs designed to present applicable concepts proved too abstract. Terms such as helicy, negentropy, and energy fields seemed difficult to understand. In a day-long workshop on the model, participants remembered being asked to "Close your eyes and breathe in the green" as they watched slides of color flash on the screen. Many nurses left asking each other, "How in the world do I use this information to plan and provide care to my clients?" One part of the orientation program was a 13-minute film explaining the definitions and principles of homeodynamics. Though it is a good film for individuals familiar with the theory, its language can be overwhelming to new employees.

In 1991, the language associated with Rogers' conceptual framework continued to be an obstacle to a smooth transition from theory to practical application. Upon review of the orientation module for nursing, we found that numerous staff were sent to clinical areas with little ability to use the model in practice. Learning the theories and principles of a conceptual model and applying the knowledge to practice requires action, participation, and commitment (Tudor, Keegan-Jones, & Bens, 1992). We realized that presenting clinical examples relevant to present nursing practice would facilitate understanding. Nurse managers were verbalizing the need for adequate theoretical preparation of new staff so that the concepts could be applied to client care immediately following the week of orientation.

Such was our challenge. The program that was characterized as difficult to implement in a clinical setting by many staff members was now changed for immediate use. The expectation was that new staff members would have the ability to apply the principles of the model to practice in the clinical setting following orientation.

STAFF ORIENTATION

To meet this expectation, it was clear that methods of introducing the model in orientation needed to be changed. Our goal was to change the introduction to Rogers' model to make it more meaningful and helpful for our staff. We planned to do this by use of participatory educational methods, use of relevant clinical examples, and simplicity of language. The importance of viewing our clients from the same nursing perspective is initially discussed with the group. This common perspective helps staff to communicate with both the client and other staff so that clients' patterns, life process variances, and priorities of care are understood.

Rogers' model is introduced by explaining that the philosophy is person-environment in its approach and helps us to view the client from this unique nursing perspective. Introduction of the principles of homeodynamics follows this explanation. Participants receive a copy of definitions within this framework to review, and make notes regarding questions and examples for further clarification.

Definitions and Clinical Examples

Unitary Human Beings.   Six small brown sandwich bags are distributed to participants. Within each bag is a piece of an action figure—two arms, two legs, one torso, and one head. Participants are instructed to take turns opening their bag, removing the contents and describing what they have found to the rest of the group. The facilitator asks additional questions: Are there any identifying marks on the body part (tattoos, additional fingers, birthmarks, jewelry, etc.)? What is the significance of these identifying marks? Describe the whole individual that this body part comes from, based on what you see.

Participants are then instructed to bring the pieces together at one table. Typically, there is laughter and amazement. We discuss how different the figure is when the whole person is viewed. We discuss the participants' descriptions of the perceived whole when based upon the viewing of one part, compared to how much more diverse the person becomes when looking at the whole. We then ask them to describe what the person is like: Is the person interested in athletics or painting? Is the person kind and considerate or cruel? They realize they have insufficient information to answer these questions about pattern manifestations of a human energy field.

What about you?, we ask. What pattern manifestations of your energy field have we seen this week as the new employee? Are you excited about a new job, anxious about being in a new clinical setting, wondering if you will fit in? There is so much more to each one of you than what you present here at work. Your human energy and environmental fields encompass your roles as mothers, fathers, daughters, sons, caretakers of family, and caregivers at work. We're afraid of a bump in the night, but respond immediately to healthcare emergencies. We are unique, diverse human beings, just as our clients are unique and diverse. We cannot stress enough the importance of treating the whole person and staying away from the cookie-cutter mentality of illness-focused care. Care must be individualized and based upon a unitary perspective of wholeness.

We then use a case study to compare and contrast the unitary perspective to the "medical model" of care. It is usually at this point that participants begin to see the significance of dealing with the whole individual and the integral role of nursing in the process.

Case Study 1. Mr. N, age 32, arrives in the emergency room complaining of pain when bearing weight on his left foot. He is barefoot, limping, and has obvious swelling and discoloration of the last three toes. He states, "I dropped a can of enchilada sauce on my foot and I can't move my small toe. Man, it hurts."

Medical model: The physician takes a history and physical, orders front and lateral x-rays of the left foot, and labs. Laboratory results are normal. Vital signs are within normal limits. A fracture of the left small toe is noted on the x-ray. Mr. N is instructed to take Tylenol for his pain and is given instructions for use of his crutches. He is given the emergency room phone number and told to call if he has increasing pain, swelling, numbness, or if his foot becomes cold to touch. He is referred to his family physician for follow-up.

Unitary nursing model: Based upon this case study, the new employees are asked to formulate additional healthcare questions that they consider important for this client, prior to his discharge. Some of the questions posed are as follows: Has Mr. N ever been in the emergency room before? If not, how anxious is he feeling in these surroundings? If so, what was his experience? Has he had an injury in the past? Does he know methods for reducing swelling and discomfort? What type of work does Mr. N do? Will he be able to move around on crutches at work? Does he need to wear a particular shoe or uniform? Does he need to stand on his feet all day? How will he get home? Did he drive himself? Is there someone who can pick him up? Does he have a car or does he usually walk? Where does he live? Will he need to climb stairs?

Staff learn that looking at the whole presents a much different picture than just treating the part that hurts. By asking these questions, the nurse learns about pattern manifestations of the client's human and environmental field and about ways to enhance deliberate mutual patterning to promote health and well-being. When clients have an opportunity to set priorities, ask questions concerning signs and symptoms that require further attention, and address issues regarding care in the home, client outcomes are improved and client and staff satisfaction increases. Case studies assist new employees in the integration of theory and practice. Through descriptions of clinical situations, some of the knowledge embedded in the expert's practice becomes visible (Benner, 1984).

Integrality and Mutual Process.   We discuss the definition of environmental field as being infinite and including anything external to a unitary human being. We ask participants to give examples of environmental pattern manifestations that promote comfort. Typically, the responses include: quiet, peaceful, sunny, warm, favorite music, family members present. We then ask them to describe the surroundings in a hospital. Responses tend to be: busy, noisy, bright lights, mechanical sounds, unfamiliar vocabulary, cold, scary.

We remind them that they are integral with the clients' environmental field. We ask them to brainstorm what they can do to pattern the surroundings to promote clients' ability to knowingly participate in change and to know that we will support their choices. Answers typically include: Listen to the client. Get back to him or her when you say you will. Turn down the lights at night. Turn down the alarm system to prevent loud, shrill noises. Encourage family participation. Do not eat at the nurses' station. Be an advocate for the patient.

We discuss that change in human beings and the environment is mutual, continuous, and unpredictable. We do not know what will happen minute to minute. The idea of energy fields is foreign to many; we remind them of electrocardiograms and electroencephalograms, which graph physiological electrical energy patterns and represent observable data that add to the continuously evolving pattern profiles of individual fields (Rogers, 1989).

Case Study 2.   To illustrate the principle of integrality and mutual process, the following story was offered. The story illustrates a method known as interpretive teaching. Nurses' experiences provide rich material for discovering shared meanings and understandings (Rittman, 1995).

Several years ago, a nurse was admitted to an area hospital for treatment of kidney stones and had an experience that changed her professional practice forever. The first day of admission was a day of left flank pain, and poking and prodding by medical staff. That night, her roommate was asleep, the room was dark, and she had just dropped off to sleep. All of a sudden, there was a loud thump as the door to the room swung open and hit the wall. The overhead lights went on, and the bright lights were blinding. A nurse shuffled in with a blanket draped across her shoulders in the form of a shawl. She was mumbling "They keep this place too cold, night after night, I just can't get warm. I'm so tired, these nights are killing me." While mumbling, she placed a blood pressure cuff on the patient's arm and pumped it up to a systolic of 200. She placed a cold stethoscope on the patient's arm, listened for her blood pressure, missed it, and pumped it up again.

The night nurse never introduced herself, never acknowledged the client's presence by saying hello. She never asked if the client had pain or offered to help her re-position. Then she shuffled her way back to the door, flipped off the lights, and closed the door with a thud. The client finally fell asleep, but at 5 A.M., a similar episode took place. And so it continued for two more nights.

On the fourth night, the client was ready for her. She figured it would be of no use to fall asleep, so she stayed awake, waiting for the first intrusion. The door opened slightly and then closed with a dull thud. Oh, here she comes again, the patient thought while laying in the darkness. She then heard soft footsteps and saw a penlight shining on her IV fluids. A voice whispered, "Oh, Ms. J, you're still awake? It's been a rough week, hasn't it?" The nurse told the client that her name was Melissa, and asked her if she was in pain. She checked her blood pressure after warming the stethoscope in her hand. She told the client that her pain medication was due in 20 minutes and she'd bring it right in. She then offered to help the client turn over, straighten out the sheets, and tuck a pillow or two behind her back. Following the medication, she adjusted the call light so that it could be reached. She placed her hand on the client's shoulder saying, "I'm right outside your door; don't hesitate to call if you need anything."

This story is presented as the experience of changing patterns of human/environmental fields. As defined by the principle of integrality, person and environment are inseparable and continuous mutual change is expected. Nurses are involved contextually in assisting clients to participate in patterning to obtain better health and well-being and to strive toward accomplishing their goals (Buczny, Speirs, & Howard, 1989).

Helicy. One can never go back. That wonderful night at your prom can never be repeated as it was, nor can you decide at age 49, that you'd prefer to be 21 again. Human beings evolve through life, carrying with them their experiences, values, and health variances. As the life process evolves, patterns change and the human and environmental fields become more diverse. Situations we face may appear to be similar to past incidents, but as experience increases, and our environmental field changes, so do we. We ask participants to think about their lives. Have they become less diverse over time? Consider the number of medications available in 1985 as compared to 1996. We struggle to maintain a sense of professionalism when our patients hand us a bottle of an unfamiliar drug. We find ourselves running to the Physician's Desk Reference. It's hard to keep up to date as life becomes more diverse.

A final example of the ever-increasing diversity and innovativeness of life may be expressed through the following illustration:

Eren is hungry. It's 4 P.M., and his mother starts to cook supper.

2 months	*Eren cries. His mother bounces him around to find out why he is crying. Is he wet? Tired? In pain? Hungry?*
11 months	*Eren cries and points to the cookie jar.*
18 months	*Eren says, "Cookie peeze."*
3 years	*Eren knows that no amount of crying, pointing, or asking politely will obtain a cookie when Mommy is cooking supper. So, he waits until Mommy has left the kitchen and then pushes a chair to the cookie jar and helps himself.*

Pattern. Pattern identifies energy fields. Life patterns reflect an individual's wholeness and uniqueness. Pattern is perceived as a single wave of energy and may be of low or high frequency. Think of blood pressure, sleep, or a hormonal cycle as rhythms that provide an index of an evolving profile. Patterns are not fixed, but change through the mutual process of human/environmental fields. Patterns are very important in assisting the nurse to understand the wholeness of unitary human beings and the uniqueness of their human/environmental fields. Think of a family's pattern during the dinner hour. Do the family members sit down, talk about the day's events, laugh over humorous incidents? Or do they eat standing up at the counter so they can finish quickly and get on to the next meeting or TV show? Or, do they eat around the TV and rarely speak to each other? How we communicate, perceive, feel, know, choose, move, and relate within our environmental field reflects our uniqueness as a diverse human being.

Unitary human beings are characterized by the capacity for abstraction and imagery, language and thought, sensation and emotion. Through these operational capacities, people are able to communicate with one another, solve difficulties, feel connected with others, and relate experience through the use of creative expression. These capabilities set us apart from other living creatures and underscore our unique nature within the cosmos.

During the initial hour of Rogerian theory, the three principles of homeodynamics are discussed and clarified. The Rogers' orientation module has evolved into a format which encourages staff participation, use of relevant clinical examples and simplicity of language.

ROGERS IN CLINICAL PRACTICE

Staff report that Rogers' model carries accountability for both client and nurse, which they enthusiastically support. Our new nursing appraisal tool helps the healthcare professional discern the degree to which personal health is valued. It identifies life process variances and appraises the unitary human being-environmental process. Staff have responded to our format for orientation: many of our hospital units have incorporated the model into their practice by including the client in the plan of care. A multidisciplinary team develops a plan from the client's perspective. The following examples provided by staff demonstrate how they apply the model in their area:

> On Psychiatry we realize we must manage the care of multiple situations. If we ignore aspects of the client's physical condition, it is more difficult to treat the psychological condition.

This nurse provided an example of a retired Marine who used alcohol excessively, in addition to being hard of hearing and arthritic. The nurse stated, "Before he retired, he had a job and could control his drinking. Now he has lost the esteem of his job, is not controlling his drinking, and his physical condition is worsening with age. His life is now more challenged and more diverse." The staff uses a multidisciplinary approach with all client care. The client and a team composed of medical, nursing, dietary, pharmacy, occupational therapy, and social work professionals plan the client's care and review its progress. (Sean Flavin, RN, BSN)

A staff nurse on the Spinal Cord Injury (SCI) unit wrote, "We did a study on the use of Therapeutic Touch and neurogenic pain in SCI patients. We did this study because of Rogers' model." Descriptive results favored the use of therapeutic touch. (G. Garcenila, RN, MS, NP)

The last example is from a staff nurse in the emergency room. She wrote, "Yesterday, I taught a homeless, disheveled, malodorous, client with chronic obstructive pulmonary disease how to use a peak flow meter and a spacer (aerochamber) with his inhalers. I had just returned from our Rogerian meeting. As I gazed at several months' accumulation of dirt under his fingernails, I hoped I could assist him to knowingly participate in his healthcare and recognize the need to improve his hygiene. Remembering that man is more than and different from the sum of his parts, it occurred to me that perhaps I should teach him how to wash his hands before expecting him to wash his spacer once a week in warm soapy water. I thought to myself, Martha would probably smile and say something like, 'the dirty nails are only one manifestation of his energy field.' So, I made a little supply kit which included his medications, inhalers, spacer, instructions, and some soap. He beamed at me like a child receiving an unexpected gift. As he left the area, he said he would wash his hands along with his spacer *every* Sunday. I felt like I had promoted the Art of Nursing that day." (Mary Newell, RN, BSN)

CONCLUSION

Nurse managers have reported an increase in the new staff members' ability to apply the model to clinical practice. Our department has also conducted a one hour program for two graduate nursing programs, at their request. Comments noted following the program were: "This is great, I finally understand the principles now," "I could never quite grasp Rogers' conceptual model and certainly couldn't understand how to apply it to a patient care setting. This has been so helpful," and, "You make it so easy—I love this model. I'm hooked on Rogers."

REFERENCES

Benner, P. (1984). *From novice to expert: Excellence and power in clinical nursing practice.* Menlo Park, CA: Addison-Wesley.

Buczny, B., Speirs, J., & Howard, Jr. (1989). Nursing care of the terminally ill client: Applying Martha Rogers' conceptual framework. *Home Health Nurse,* 7(4), 13-18.

Falco, S. M., & Lobo, M. L. (1995). *Nursing theories: The base for professional nursing practice* (4th ed.). Norwalk, CT: Appleton & Lange.

Fitch, M., Roger, M., Ross, E., Shea, H., Smith, I., & Tucker, D. (1991). Developing a plan to evaluate the use of nursing conceptual frameworks. *Canadian Journal of Nursing Administration, 4,* 22-28.

Heggie, J. R., Schoenmehl, P. A., Chang, M. K., & Grieco, C. (1989). Selection and implementation of Dr. Martha Rogers' nursing conceptual model in an acute care setting. *Clinical Nurse Specialist, 3*(3), 143-147.

Malinski, V. N. (1993). Therapeutic touch: The view from Rogerian nursing science. *Visions: The Journal of Rogerian Nursing Science, 1*(1), 45-54.

Rittman, M. (1995). Storytelling: An innovative approach to staff development. *Journal of Nursing Staff Development, 11*(1), 15-19.

Rogers, M. (1989). Questions for Dr. Martha E. Rogers: Dr. Rogers' answer. *Rogerian Nursing Science News, 1*(3), 6.

Tudor, C. A., Keegan-Jones, L., & Bens, E. M. (1992). Implementing Rogers' science based nursing practice in a pediatric nursing service setting. In M. Madrid & E. A. M. Barrett (Eds.), *Rogers scientific art of nursing practice* (pp. 305-322). New York: NLN Press.

23

The Practice of Nursing from a Unitary Perspective

Jeanie Gold

*T*he changing face of healthcare has created undulating waves in the practice of nursing. Examples abound: reduced length of hospital stays, expanding complexity of client care needs, challenges posed by managed care, fewer available nursing jobs in acute care settings, institutional budget reductions resulting in greater numbers of people that individual nurses are caring for, growing consumer demand for natural and/or holistic approaches to healthcare, and so forth. These changes have created an opportunity for nurses to examine their current practice and define new innovative ways to deliver nursing care. Contemporary healthcare realities have left some nurses to examine their methods of practice, wondering exactly how they can honor their professional responsibilities and, at the same time, feel good about the work they do.

Given the many new challenges we all face, the students and nurses that I work with often question the possibility of being able to care for "the whole person." Practicing nursing from a unitary perspective and viewing the person as a whole is an important aspect of finding meaning, value, and satisfaction in a nurse's work. Utilizing a unitary framework in nursing seems crucial in the process of distinguishing the uniqueness of nursing practice.

Though the foundation of professional nursing is recognized as holistic in origin (Nightengale, 1946), it was Martha Rogers (1970, 1994) who defined nursing as an organized body of knowledge and paved the way for the practice of nursing as a scientific art. Rogers forged a new way of thinking that is unique to nursing.

Rogers' Science of Unitary Human Beings is a revolutionary nursing paradigm that presents a new way of thinking about people and their world. It was not "derived from one or more of the basic sciences," but emerged as a new product "arrived at by the creative synthesis of facts and ideas" (Rogers, 1992, p. 28). The principles and theories derived from Rogerian science present a new worldview that describes the irreducible wholeness of people and their universe. This unitary perspective must be articulated in language that does not present a fragmented view.

It has been proposed that Rogerian science and Rogers' principles of integrality, helicy, and resonancy are congruent with concepts of new physics and with Bohm's theory of Wholeness and the Implicate Order (Carboni, 1995). Bohm (1980) recognized that ordinary language does not reflect "unbroken wholeness" or one-ness and that "a new mode of language" is necessary to accurately portray the unitary nature of reality (p. 30).

Practicing nursing from a unitary perspective requires that one develop a nonlinear, irreducible way of looking at people and their environment. It is nothing short of learning a new language and a new way of thinking. The language used to communicate a unitary perspective must not be causal, fragmented, or reductionist.

Considering that ordinary, everyday, three-dimensional language is viewed as causal, linear, and particulate in nature (Bohm, 1980; Capra, 1982, 1991), many commonly used words are not useful when identifying, describing, and clarifying unitary concepts. Rogers recognized the difficulty of finding the "right word" when speaking or writing about the Science of Unitary Human Beings. She, too, was not always satisfied with her chosen word(s) but, at that relative time, it was the best she could do (Madrid, M., personal communication, June 15, 1996). An example is the updating of her definitions. Four-dimensional was updated to multidimensional, but still did not capture the essence of what Rogers meant. Her "Aha!" came at 3:00 AM one morning when she "knew that *pandimensional* was the right word" (Rogers, 1994, p. 4).

It is the responsibility of educators to clarify new paradigm thinking, related concepts and vernacular, and to facilitate the application to practice. Unless the educational approach is understandable to the learner, it seems unlikely that the Science of Unitary Human Beings will be widely used in nursing practice. Admittedly, there is immense challenge in attempting to clarify and apply Rogers' nursing model while avoiding language that is causal, linear, and reductionist. The following is offered with this challenge in mind.

PRACTICING NURSING FROM A UNITARY PERSPECTIVE

In this chapter, Rogers' Science of Unitary Human Beings is being applied to the scientific art of nursing practice. Two personal experiences are offered as examples. Names and other identifying information have been changed to ensure confidentiality.

To assist in the application of Rogers' model in nursing practice, the following guidelines are provided:

1. Nursing is the study of unitary human beings in continuous mutual process with their irreducible environments.
2. Nursing practice is the art of applying nursing knowledge.
3. Humans are recognized as unitary beings, meaning that they are inseparable/irreducible.
4. Nursing care of unitary human beings is understood to be universally applicable in any situation or setting.
5. Nursing care is synonymous with "whole person" care, regardless of realities in the healthcare system or changes and challenges imposed by it.

Valentino

Valentino was 82 years old and was admitted to the hospital with the medical diagnoses of sepsis, atrial fibrillation, and pemphigus. From a Rogerian perspective, these physical manifestations are recognized as life-patterning difficulties. Within the Science of Unitary Human Beings, disease is not seen as an isolated aspect of a person's life experience. Rather, it provides a holographic glimpse of a person's human energy field pattern. Focusing on a particular medical diagnosis or on related signs and symptoms is a fragmented view of a person. This reductionist approach denies the reality of the indivisible wholeness of human beings who are in mutual process with their ever-changing environmental field.

In reality, there are no separate parts. "There is no mind, no body, no spirit, only the inherent unity of who we are" (Barrett, 1994, p. 77).

Though separating a person into parts may be helpful in simplifying the learning process, in actuality, this particulate approach is not a true reflection of the wholeness of human beings. According to Koplowitz (1984), "the process of naming or measuring pulls that which is named out of reality, which itself is not nameable or measurable" (p. 288).

The behavioral manifestations of Valentino's energy field characterized a pattern of passion and independence. He expressed himself loudly and passionately, with the intent to be heard and understood. He was adamant about caring for himself and maintaining his independence in spite of the weakness, exhaustion, and challenges that his medical condition posed.

The diffuse pemphigus wounds that covered Valentino's body continuously oozed a malodorous drainage and were infected with methicillin-resistant staphylococcus aureus (MRSA). Valentino had a great deal of pain and discomfort, and he struggled continuously to move into a less painful position. Despite medication, his pain was unrelenting.

The resonating pattern of Valentino's inseparable human and environmental fields was not always harmonious. This was especially evident when his wife and daughter visited. These visits usually lasted only five to ten minutes, occurred only once or twice a week, and each visit was marked by loud yelling and agitated gesturing.

Following a particularly volatile visit, Valentino was found alone, kneeling at his bedside, yelling, thrashing his arms, and refusing to be touched. Recognizing and respecting Valentino's pattern manifestations of agitation and emotional upset, I knowingly participated in changing our mutual environmental field pattern by utilizing silent, active listening (deliberate/intentional mutual patterning). My intention for doing this was to foster conscious trust. Using nodding and caring facial expressions, I acknowledged and validated the importance of Valentino's words and the feelings he expressed.

For a while, what we did was to simply "be" in one another's presence. Time and space seemed to be nonexistent and we transcended conventional, ordinary communication. In that quiet, pandimensional moment, neither of us spoke and we seemed to sense the rhythm of each other's humanness. There was a heightened awareness of the integral mutual process of our human/environmental energy fields. Recognizing Valentino as being integral with my environmental energy field and myself as being integral with his, I knowingly participated with Valentino in his flow of life. I was intentionally coming from a pandimensional place of gentleness and unconditional caring, which exemplified being attuned to the changing rhythms and pattern of my energy field.

Since Valentino did not speak English, a translator provided a wonderful avenue for him to express himself. He spoke, yelled, and cursed for a considerable length of time. Gradually, his words were spoken more slowly and softly, and he permitted me to assist him off his knees and back to bed. I stayed with Valentino and he shared his thoughts and feelings with me. Valentino expressed anger and frustration about the chronic nature of his medical condition and the experience of repeatedly being hospitalized over the past few years. He struggled with what he described as "unbearable pain" and feeling "isolated, untouchable, and like an unwanted burden" to his family.

I perceived manifestations of Valentino's receptiveness and willingness to participate in the process of healing and for me to use touch as a caring, healing therapeutic modality. Mindful of the tenderness of Valentino's diffuse wounds, I spoke with him (via a translator) about Therapeutic Touch (Krieger, 1979) and how it has been known to promote calmness and relaxation and to help soothe pain. Though Valentino was unfamiliar with the field patterning modality of Therapeutic Touch, he asked very few questions and readily agreed to receive it.

Recognizing the integrality and mutual processing of our energy fields, I focused my intent to help Valentino, assumed a meditative state of awareness (Meehan, 1990) and I gave him a Therapeutic Touch treatment. Shortly after the treatment, a look of peacefulness transformed Valentino's face. His respiratory rate and rhythm slowed and deepened, and he fell asleep.

Somewhere in a place beyond words, Valentino touched my heart and allowed me to touch his. As Valentino knowingly participated in our shared healing process, I was aware of a resonating pattern I define as love, emerging from the mutual processing of our human/environmental fields. I will never forget Valentino. I carry with me a deep knowing that my life has been profoundly changed by my experience with Valentino and I continue to feel his pandimensional presence in my life.

Victoria

Victoria was 89 years old and was admitted to the hospital with the medical diagnosis of severe cerebral vascular accident (CVA). The physical manifestations of Victoria's energy field were extensive paralysis and expressive aphasia. During Victoria's hospital stay, she never received any visitors and it was unclear as to whether or not she had a family. Prior to her admission, Victoria was living in a nursing home and participated in independent self-care activities of daily living.

When I first met Victoria, she was lying in bed, restless, vigorously rocking her head, making moaning sounds, and crying softly. The anguish and frustration she was experiencing was perceived by these manifestations and by her tensely contorted facial expression. Recognizing that "pattern is grasped only in and through its expressions" (Cowling, 1990,

p. 53), I appraised her physical and behavioral manifestations to be expressions of Victoria's energy field pattern.

According to Malinski (1993), "the nurse experiences her/his integrality with the environmental field by assuming a meditative, pandimensional form of awareness" (p. 52). For a short while, I remained at Victoria's bedside in a quiet, reflective, meditative state. My intention was to capture the unitary wholeness of Victoria and to knowingly participate in the integral mutual processing of our environmental energy fields.

I introduced myself to Victoria, briefly explained the reason for my visit, and lowered my face to a level equal to hers. I softly touched Victoria's arm and gently took her hand in mine. I spontaneously felt a strong resonating pattern I define as love, as I focused my intent on helping Victoria. Within moments, Victoria established eye contact with me. She became very still and emanated a resonating pattern that I perceived as harmony and peacefulness. As Victoria relaxed, the pattern of her breathing became quiet and restful. Her facial expression changed and she "glowed" with an ethereal beauty. Victoria looked into my eyes, turned the unaffected side of her mouth upward and gave me an asymmetric smile. I appraised these manifestations to be an expression of Victoria's awareness of her knowing participation in the healing process.

I, too, was aware of the integrality of our human/environmental field process as I experienced a deep sense of quietness and peacefulness. In that pandimensional moment, Victoria and I transcended the usual manner of communication and it seemed that space and time did not exist. There are no words that I know of to describe what I experienced. I was aware of a soothing, all-encompassing white light, a sense of oneness, and a feeling of sacred presence with Victoria. I sensed that she, too, had this experience. As with Valentino, I continue to feel Victoria's pandimensional presence in my life.

The healing process that Victoria and I knowingly participated in is one of the most profound experiences I have ever had. It served to transform my professional practice, to enhance my personal growth, and has contributed immensely to the joy I feel in my work as a nurse. This mutual process with Victoria awakened me to a sense of awe regarding the sacred moments that may be experienced as a nurse, when caring for unitary human beings.

CONCLUSION

It is more crucial than ever that nurses clearly understand and identify the uniqueness of nursing. In light of the ongoing upheaval and "restructuring" occurring in the healthcare industry, it is important for nurses to keep focused on their phenomenon of concern that is "people and the world they live in" (Rogers, 1992).

As healthcare roles and responsibilities continue to shift and evolve, it is essential that nurses be educated about and have the ability to articulate what distinguishes their science from that of other healthcare providers. Not only will this clarification serve to guide the vision, purpose, and practice of nursing, it is also integral to nurses finding meaning, value, and satisfaction in their work.

Martha Rogers has identified nursing as a unique and independent discipline, one that is not defined by summarizing knowledge from other fields. Rogerian science identifies a distinctive body of knowledge that distinguishes the uniqueness of nursing as a basic science, "whose aim is to promote health and well-being for all persons wherever they are" (Malinski, 1994, pp. 203–204). As we respond to the "call for participation in a radical change of healthcare (Barrett, 1994, p. 62), Rogers' new worldview of irreducible wholeness and a unitary nursing model will best serve nurses as we move toward the 21st century.

REFERENCES

Barrett, E. A. M. (1994). Rogerian scientists, artists, revolutionaries. In M. Madrid & E. A. M. Barrett (Eds.), *Rogers' scientific art of nursing practice* (pp. 61–80). New York: NLN Press.

Bohm, D. (1980). *Wholeness and the implicate order.* New York: Routledge.

Capra, F. (1982). *The turning point: Science, society, and the rising culture.* New York: Simon & Schuster.

Capra, F. (1991). *The tao of physics: An exploration of the parallels between modern physics and eastern mysticism* (3rd ed.). Boston: Shambhala.

Carboni, J. (1995). Enfolding health-as-wholeness-and-harmony: A theory of Rogerian nursing practice. *Nursing Science Quarterly, 8*(2), 71–78.

Cowling, W. R. (1990). A template for unitary pattern-based nursing practice. In E. A. M. Barrett (Ed.), *Visions of Rogers' science-based nursing* (pp. 45–65). New York: NLN Press.

Koplowitz, H. (1984). A projection beyond Piaget's formal operational stage: A general system stage and a unitary stage. In M. L. Commons, F. A. Richards, & C. Armon (Eds.), *Beyond formal operations: Late adolescent and adult cognitive development* (pp. 272–295). New York: Praeger.

Krieger, D. (1979). *The therapeutic touch: How to use your hands to heal.* Englewood Cliffs, NJ: Prentice-Hall.

Malinski, V. (1993). Therapeutic touch: The view from Rogerian nursing science. *Visions: The Journal of Rogerian Nursing Science,* 45–54.

Malinski, V. (1994). Highlights in the evolution of nursing science: Emergence of the science of unitary human beings. In V. Malinski & E. A. M. Barrett (Eds.), *Martha E. Rogers: Her life and her work* (pp. 197-204). Philadelphia: F.A. Davis.

Meehan, T. (1990). The science of unitary human beings and theory based practice: Therapeutic touch. In E. A. M. Barrett (Ed.), *Visions of Rogers' science-based nursing* (pp. 67-81). New York: NLN Press.

Nightengale, F. (1946). *Notes on nursing: What it is, and what it is not.* Philadelphia: F.A. Davis.

Rogers, M. (1970). *An introduction to the theoretical basis of nursing.* Philadelphia: F.A. Davis.

Rogers, M. (1990). Nursing: Science of unitary, irreducible human beings: Update 1990. In E. A. M. Barrett (Ed.), *Visions of Rogers' science-based nursing* (pp. 5-11). New York: NLN Press.

Rogers, M. (1992). Nursing science and the space age. *Nursing Science Quarterly, 5*(1), 27-34.

Rogers, M. (1994). The science of unitary human beings: Current perspectives. *Nursing Science Quarterly, 7*(1), 33-35.

24

Practicing Medicine in the Nineties with an Emphasis on the Unitary Perspective of Patient Care

Jeffrey L. Gold

*T*reating the patient as a whole becomes more of a challenge as one goes deeper and deeper into a managed care environment. Throughout medical school and residency, physicians are taught the fundamentals of anatomy, physiology, and pathology and, over the years, these are interwoven into clinical experiences. We integrate this knowledge and experience in practice with the hope of treating each patient as a complete being, realizing all the while that there is more beyond the diagnosis and treatment of their varied conditions. As our patients relate their health concerns and difficulties to us, in addition to being nonjudgmental listeners, we must also honor the fact that, while perhaps unsaid, there is an equally important emotional/spiritual connection coincident with their condition that we must also appreciate. Patients are viewed quite differently from a unitary perspective. This perspective should be the essence of what practicing medicine is about.

Over the years, by working with Rogerian nurses, I have been introduced to the Science of Unitary Human Beings. Although the language and terms at times seem hard to grasp, the message that unitary human beings are "irreducible wholes" and that healthcare providers cannot understand the wholeness of a person by appraising them in parts is clear. I have seen how the delivery of nursing care from a unitary perspective has made a difference in patient outcome. I was involved in the care of Carlos, the client that Mary Madrid described in a case study to illustrate the use of Rogers' model in practice (Madrid & Woods Smith, 1994).

Carlos was admitted on multiple occasions to the intensive care unit, comatose and with a toxic level of alcohol. He required intubation and went through several days of nearly uncontrollable seizure activity. Upon awakening, he would be agitated and extremely combative. The intensive care nursing staff often feared physical harm because of Carlos' strength. This, coupled with his hallucinatory manifestations of alcohol withdrawal, made Carlos' overall care a tremendous challenge. The complex nature of each of his admissions provided me with a smorgasbord of medical management and technical procedures that a medical intern revels in. I also became well versed in the "stabilize and transfer" doctrine that most inner city medical center intensive care units must conform to.

It was during my final rotation in the ICU as a medical intern that Carlos was once again admitted with his all too familiar, and at this point frustrating, scenario. His usual regimen of respiratory insufficiency requiring ventilator support, fluid resuscitation, seizure control, and correction of his multiple metabolic abnormalities ensued. It was during this admission that his almost permanently assigned nurse, Mary Madrid, and I sat down and had several discussions about "innovative ways" of dealing with Carlos' present situation. Some of the terms used certainly were alien (pattern appraisals, human field patterning), but the overall concept of approaching Carlos' care from a unitary perspective was fascinating.

The degree of Carlos' physical and verbal combativeness post-extubation required that he be assigned one of the "quiet rooms" in the intensive care unit. These were freestanding rooms with solid walls and a door, as opposed to the generic curtaining that is usually found between beds in an ICU. I was able to obtain a radio from the staff on-call room, which was placed at Carlos' bedside and tuned to a soothing FM station. A close shave was rendered with extreme caution due to his coagulopathy, and a thorough cleansing of his scalp hair and body was administered.

Early extubation was carried out and a mirror was held in front of Carlos. He was able to stroke his closely shaven face and run his fingers through his free-flowing hair, which was usually matted down and stuck to his head. His traditional four-point restraints were at the ready, but did not need to be implemented this time. Just as it was mesmerizing for me to see what was transpiring, it was even more powerful for Carlos to gain insight as to what was happening to him and his immediate world. The therapeutic modalities that Mary Madrid initiated made an astounding difference in his well-being. His power of self-healing was enhanced as he knowingly participated in change.

We transferred Carlos out of ICU to a nursing unit on a medical floor. He was quite receptive to the ancillary support teams that were available in the hospital—social services and pastoral care. We did have several other "meetings" during my years as a resident and he made a gradual transition through a 12-step program. He also became involved in religious activities. I no longer provide his medical care, but to this day, when I see him, he always has his Bible.

This experience with Carlos was profound. It opened up a new way of viewing patients and caring for them. It went beyond the medical model of pathology and disease and made a difference in "patient outcome." It was not until years later that I could appreciate my role and my participation in the patterning process that enhanced Carlos' self-healing power and his progress toward reaching his goals. This experience was one of many in which a light bulb was turned on, illuminating new pathways to enable me to further understand the uniqueness of human beings and their unitary wholeness and how I, as a physician, could synthesize this knowledge, acquire meaning from it, and use it creatively in my practice of medicine and in my personal growth.

But how do healthcare providers deliver care from a unitary perspective in a managed care environment with enormous constraints that must be faced on a daily basis? How can we offer our patients the most appropriate care when each and every step is wrought with mountains of paperwork, phone calls, voice mail recordings, and computer generated approvals or denials?

Healthcare, as it is presented in its current state, is supposed to be "problem oriented." The healthcare institutions that currently control the bulk of our hospital and office practices today expect the provider to address only the "problem" that the patient presents with and forget that there is a whole, complete being lying on our examination table. Glass (1996) states that:

> In the new era of cost controls and managed care, the incentive to do more that was present in fee-for-service has shifted dramatically to the incentive to do less. The less usually includes less time spent with each patient, a fundamental threat to establishing a good patient-physician

relationship. Additional threats in capitated or managed care settings in-
clude loss of physician autonomy to make clinical decisions in the best
interests of patients, loss of patient trust, loss of continuity of relation-
ships and adversarial and ethical problems with financial incentives to
limit care. (p. 148)

One of the most difficult aspects of providing healthcare from a unitary perspective is to arrive at the point where the patient, as well as the
insurance companies, are able to come to the realization that "chief complaints" cannot be "cured" with a ten-day supply of antibiotic therapy or
analgesics, but require not only acute, but long-term and, at times, life-
long, behavioral health patterning, therapeutic modalities. At least 25
percent of the patients in a primary care practice present with emotional
problems such as anxiety, depression, or drug or alcohol abuse (Marwick,
1996). It takes more than a few generic office visits for the physician and
patient to establish a sense of mutual trust.

The patient/physician relationship is the center of medicine. It should
be a "moral enterprise grounded in a covenant of trust" (Glass, 1996,
p. 148). This moral enterprise encompasses mutual trust and respect. The
physician should not be in a controlling and dominant position, with the
patient being submissive and obedient. Rather, the approach to care
should be a mutual process of exploration and decision making, with the
patient being an active participant in this process. The physician uncon-
ditionally respects the ultimate decision that the patient makes and com-
passionately assists and supports his or her chosen plan of care. Consider
the following experiences with patients that I have seen in my practice.
Their names have been changed to provide anonymity.

Trudy

Trudy, a 22-year-old white female came to my office for her initial visit accompanied by her mother. She weighed 76 pounds and had a cachectic
appearance. It was clear when speaking with the patient and her mother
that Trudy had a long-standing eating disorder that was never adequately
addressed. After taking an indepth history and performing a physical examination, I discussed the need for psychiatric therapy with this young
woman. In Rogerian terms, she would benefit from health patterning.

Rather than being able to tell the patient that, in my opinion, a specific
referral would be best suited for her health needs, I had to tell her that,
for her to be referred for counseling and psychiatric therapy, she would
have to call the 800 number printed on the back of her insurance mem-
bership card so that she would be guaranteed coverage. What this would

not guarantee was the appropriateness of the computer-generated referral she would receive or the quality of the therapist whose name she would be given. This was not a caring and compassionate approach for a potentially life-threatening disorder that could change drastically with the appropriate attention and the patient's involvement in creating change.

Trudy and I discussed the options of care available ranging from the "spin the wheel and hope for the best approach" that was outlined on her health provider card, to the more humanistic approach of discussing the various eating disorder specialists in the area. We also considered a long-term "in-house program" that may or may not be deemed "medically necessary" by her insurance providers.

Wanda

Wanda, a 46-year-old black female came to my office for a routine follow-up visit for management of her hypertension. Her pressure reading was 170/110 and she looked visibly upset. Recognizing that something other than her high blood pressure was contributing to her emotional state, we discussed the underlying dynamics of her distress.

I learned that the essence of her emotional turmoil was that a family member had died and she was receiving pressure to attend the funeral services. After several minutes, the patient tearfully revealed that the person who recently passed away had molested her when she was a child. After discussing in more detail that a time for healing was long overdue, the invariable question came up as to whether or not her healthcare coverage would be financially accountable for any bills incurred in addressing this health need. Certainly, her blood pressure could be controlled with further modification of her medication, but equally important was the need to address other aspects of her well-being. Wanda chose to seek guidance from trusted members of her church community. I supported her decision.

Helen

Helen, a 33-year-old black, female nurse with a history of hypertension and polycystic kidney disease presented on a Friday afternoon with a sudden excruciating headache. The patient was keenly aware of the incidence of berry aneurysms in people with polycystic kidney disease. When we made an effort to get approval for neural imaging of the patient, we were told that it would have to wait until Monday since the medical director would not be available for the rest of the weekend. When I relayed this to the patient, who was in a state of deep anxiety, she converted to near hysteria.

Recognizing that the time it takes to get approval or to appeal a denial many times alters the final outcome of the patient's clinical course, I simply told the patient we were going to get the test that afternoon. If we could not get approval for compensation of the exam, the office would pay for it. I felt at this point that her presentation could be potentially life-threatening. I also recognized that her experience of fear and anxiety was important. She probably envisioned herself facing the worst possible health scenario. Fortunately, her scan was negative, allowing us all to be collectively relieved.

SUMMARY

In the cases presented, I broke several cardinal rules of managed care by practicing from a unitary perspective. First of all, I addressed more than the task at hand. Trudy was being seen for the physical manifestations of her eating disorder and Wanda had come for evaluation of her blood pressure. Second, in viewing the patient as a whole, I took the time to notice that there were clearly other pattern manifestations that identified specific health needs. Third, I ordered diagnostic tests without prior approval from the insurance company. Within the context of the patient/physician relationship, we may be able to mutually *define the problem* at hand. The difficulty arises in reaching a solution that best fits the patient as a whole being, a solution that comes from the heart, not one that comes from a computer-generated, laminated list of accepted clinical pathways that is circulated by many of the large healthcare organizations. In my fifteen years of private practice, I have never found it impossible to offer patient care in a holistic manner. Nor have I been unable to honor and respect the healthcare choices that patients make.

James

James was a 54-year-old white male diagnosed with carcinoma of the prostate. After numerous conversations with him outlining the various treatment options, his final choice was to begin homeopathic therapy and rely on his strong spiritual beliefs and guidance. I told him that although my personal choice may have been different, I would honor and respect his chosen pathway. We have worked together for two years giving each other mutual guidance. There has been no evidence of further spread of his disease. His option was the right one for him simply because *he chose it.* Managed care however, for the most part, has been unable to fathom this dimension of patient care and self-care orientated wellness.

The unfortunate reality of most managed healthcare systems is that the individuals in this system have no concept of the patient in his or her wholeness. They are only aware of what type of policy the patient has, what kind of coverage is permitted, and what kind of testing is allowed. The people with the decision-making power are disassociated from the patients for whom they are making these decisions.

Nancy

Nancy, a 29-year-old white female, recently underwent a lung transplant. She was doing well on triple immunotherapy following her surgery. Nancy experienced excessive menstrual bleeding, then became clinically jaundiced. She presented with a hemoglobin of 5.0 and a bilirubin of 7.2. Within hours of her hospitalization, I received a call from the case manager of her insurance company wanting to know if the hospital admission was indeed warranted.

I explained the whole scenario and was told that she would give me approval for a 24-hour stay. I explained that, even under the best of conditions, this type of presentation would require more than a one-day hospitalization. Given the fact that the patient was immunocompromised and had just had major thoracic surgery, it was more than just a standard admission for a workup and treatment of anemia and jaundice.

I held fast to my position that blood transfusions, hysterectomy, cholecystectomy, and cyclosporine toxicity needed to be dealt with in a special way, and that the focus of concern should be on the patient and not the financial aspect of care. Fortunately, Nancy's outcome was successful in terms of her treatment and response. She was, however, partially responsible financially for the necessary days that she remained in the hospital that were denied by her insurance company.

NURSE CASE MANAGERS

Imagine how much better it would have been for the insurance company to view Nancy and her health needs from a unitary perspective. What a difference this would have made! Managed healthcare systems could have "Nurse Case Managers" present on hospital sites on a scheduled basis, as opposed to "spot visits" for "problem cases." These visits invariably generate a phone call by the case manager in the middle of hectic office hours. The presario, "If the doctor does not get on the phone, the patient may be financially accountable for his or her hospital stay, and all the healthcare providers may be denied reimbursement" is given.

The title "case manager" would take on a different meaning. The intent would be to act as an advocate for the patient, rather than take away the patient's right to be autonomous and to make choices in his or her healthcare. I suggest that case managers accompany the physician on rounds and actually see patients. Talk to them, explore their hopes and fears, listen to the choices they have made or are making, appraise them as whole human beings and then decide how many days of reimbursement they are entitled to receive. It would also be helpful to have medical directors who are accessible by phone (as we are expected to be) for dialogue regarding "problem" cases.

PRACTICING FROM A UNITARY PERSPECTIVE

Attempting to practice medicine from a unitary perspective has been a self-learning process. There are so many complementary resources available. Unfortunately, there is currently little place for them in the acceptable structure of today's healthcare delivery system.

We are, however, beginning to see some changes. There are several medical centers in the United States that have begun to practice "integrated medicine" (Thomson, 1996, p. 98). In this atmosphere, traditional medicine is practiced in conjunction with complementary, alternative care. Allopathic, homeopathic, naturopathic holistic healers work for the mutual benefit of total patient care, and some insurance carriers are recognizing the utility (and at times, money-saving aspect) that such multi-faceted care offers. The use of modalities such as relaxation techniques, meditation, guided imagery, Therapeutic Touch, and various types of hands-on healing have unlimited potential in dealing with patients' health needs. It is possible that these therapeutic modalities would dramatically reduce the need for various allopathic preparations and would play an important role in such health situations as dealing with daily stress, or patients' pre- and post-operative emotional needs. A large percentage of work-related absences and poor job performance, as well as low job satisfaction are often stress-related and need to be dealt with on a very personalized level.

If the practice of medicine continues in a purely linear fashion, it will become more difficult for physicians to break down illusionary barriers and open themselves to the complementary aspects of disease treatment and wellness care. I had the opportunity to experience this on a personal level several years ago and I was "converted."

I was scheduled for a resection of the head of my humerus, with the extent of the surgery and pathology being unknown. A great deal of anxiety immediately ensued. The situation was intensified by the degree of pain that I was experiencing on a daily basis. Fortunately, my spouse, a holistic nurse familiar with the Rogerian Science of Unitary Human Beings, began to work with me on a regular basis. With hands-on healing work and guided meditation, coupled with relaxation therapy, I was able to deal with the reality of the situation on a completely different dimension. My panic quickly dissipated and my pain was significantly reduced. At the time of my surgery, I required absolutely no preoperative medications. Postoperatively, I went from a morphine drip to homeopathic remedies administered by my spouse.

Adopting the approach of participating in the process of health patterning and choosing to use my potential for healing was a memorable, significant experience. Instead of everything focusing on the technical aspects of the procedure, I was viewed and cared for as a unitary whole. *All* my needs were dealt with. Addressing my needs from this perspective must have eliminated at least one day of hospital stay and further benefited my insurance company since there was no need for any preoperative antianxiety or postoperative analgesic medication.

I now incorporate many of these techniques into my own practice. I am able to confidently offer referrals to practitioners in the area who can offer alternative, complementary services.

As a physician, practicing medicine from a unitary perspective is a way of being that emanates from a new worldview of people and their universe. This view urges me to go beyond what our present system offers in order to deliver care in a manner that acknowledges and addresses the wholeness of human beings.

Marwick (1996) quotes several physicians who spoke at the 1996 Fourth International Congress of Behavioral Medicine. Barr Taylor, immediate past president of the Society of Behavioral Medicine, stated that "Physicians take care of acute situations, but not the long term. What we are focusing on are lifestyle issues and interventions that might extend to 5 years" (p. 1145). David Sobel, director of patient education and health promotion at Kaiser Permanente Medical, Northern California Region, said that "cost effectiveness is not the bottom line—health improvement is." He further states that "Quality of life measures are now being valued as important outcome measures. Since our interventions are often aimed at the level of how people perceive themselves, we should be able to demonstrate a high payoff" . . . (p. 1145). Edward Wagner, director for health services at the Group Health Cooperative of Puget Sound in Seattle, "reported on experience with programs of behavioral medicine in influencing dietary changes and smoking cessation and encouraging participation in mammographic screening" (p. 1145).

I am learning that what these physicians are saying is what Rogerian nurses have been doing! To these nurses, "health patterning," "human field image," "power as knowing participation in change" are household words. As primary care providers, physicians must participate in creating a renaissance of compassion and caring. We must promote a view of human wholeness in the delivery of healthcare and innovatively structure the system so that the patient has the freedom and opportunity to make choices and participate in change.

REFERENCES

Glass, R. (1996, January 10). The patient-physician relationship. JAMA focuses on the center of medicine. *Journal of the American Medical Association, 275*(2), 147-148.

Madrid, M., & Woods Smith, D. (1994). Becoming literate in the science of unitary human beings. In M. Madrid & E. A. M. Barrett (Eds.), *Rogers' scientific art of nursing practice* (pp. 339-354). New York: NLN Press.

Marwick, C. (1996, April 17). Managed care may feature behavioral medicine. *Journal of the American Medical Association, 275*(11), 1144-1146.

Thomson, B. (1996, March/April). The medical revolution. *Natural Health, 26,* 98-103.

25

The Scientific Art
of Medical Practice

Steven Field

*P*andimensionality? Resonancy, helicy, and integrality? Irreducible human beings?

Oh, sure. Right.

To most physicians what possible relevance can these concepts have to the practice of medicine today? How do we as physicians integrate these principles into practice to promote health and well-being? What is the nature of, and the role of, Rogerian science in the current medical environment of high biotechnology, and what will its role be in the newly emerging and new corporatized healthcare system, a system wherein, as never before, time is money, and money, time? It would seem more than mildly difficult to reconcile two such seemingly mutually exclusive phenomena as the Science of Unitary Human Beings and the science of medicine as it has traditionally been taught in American medical schools.

But are the two really so far apart? The thesis of this discussion is that in fact they are not so antipodal, that they are rather integral and (or should be) coexistent. Physicians may not recognize some of the behaviors they

267

manifest by the Rogerian terms, but these same behaviors form the very underpinnings of the successful practice of medicine. And as our technology advances and computerized information systems and databases, as well as pressures from managed care companies, continue to revolutionize the delivery of healthcare, we as physicians are offered the opportunity to examine some of the aspects of our roles as healers. Rogers' Science of Unitary Human Beings affords an excellent paradigm for this re-examination.

Like many other disciplines, medicine is a combination of science and art. The science consists of the body of knowledge which comprises the discipline, knowledge both known and as yet unknown. This knowledge is codified into textbooks, taught in lecture halls, transmitted to students and house officers on ward rounds, and ultimately incorporated into the repertoires of succeeding generations of physicians, that is brought to bear on a daily basis in the treatment of sick patients and the prevention of disease in healthy ones. This repertoire is marked by constant fluidity, as new ideas arise and new treatments are developed and implemented. In fact, the fluidity is perhaps its most important characteristic; the physician who allows his or her database to become petrified is of little use to anyone. The science of medicine, the study of the pathology, prevention, and treatment of disease, is medicine's unique phenomenon of concern.

However, the practice of medicine also involves another aspect, the art of healing. How does healing occur outside of the realm of medical science? It occurs in many ways, most of which we may not think of as being part of medicine at all. When a mother holds a child who has skinned his knee, and comforts him, and kisses the knee, the child immediately calms down and stops crying—this is healing, as sure as mercurochrome and band-aids. A patient comes into my office with an upper respiratory infection (URI), with low-grade fever, coryza, clear phlegm, sneezing, and coughing; when I examine her and find no evidence of bacterial infection, I explain that she has a simple URI and she needs bedrest, fluids, and some nonprescription remedies. The patient often says to me on her way out of the office, "Thanks for seeing me, Doctor; I feel better already"; that, too, is healing, and that healing has little to do with medical science. That healing is about mutual respect and understanding and the physician's role as a facilitator in the patient's participation in the process of healing. On the front lines of medical care, the terminology is unimportant; we can call it patterning the environment, we can call it allowing for participation in change, we can call it a mutual field process—so long as we *do* it. This caring aspect of healing, as Rogers (1994) noted, is a requirement of all health professionals.

Healing is the art of medicine. It is the way in which healthcare providers recognize their inherent integrality with patients, allowing for mutual process to occur between them. It is not a god-process, nor is it a friendship, though it must have qualities resonant of both. It is not about test tubes and clinical trails, or bugs and drugs. It is the way in which the knowledge that comprises medical science is put to use in clinical practice, the effector of medicine. If medical science is a brand-new, high-tech, fully-loaded automobile, the art of medicine is Driver's Ed. Driver's Ed can be taught . . . Can the art of medicine be taught? Yes, it can.

Compassion cannot be taught, any more than love can be taught; there must be an experiential aspect to learning these emotions. However, a system can be set up, standardized, and communicated—taught—to students that fosters understanding of patients and that lays the foundation for the experiencing of such emotion and its assimilation into the student's clinical practice. This system would not simply teach about caring; caring is necessary, but far from sufficient. This system is a tool to enable the physician to become involved in all aspects of healing, of using medical science and medical art as a means toward ultimate wellness and restitution of health. To paraphrase the title of Madrid and Barrett's (1994) publication, this would be the scientific art of medical practice, and it will have to take its place beside the other courses in medical school, for in the coming brave new world of healthcare, healing will become more and more important, and healing cannot occur in most cases without the art of medicine.

The art of medical practice not only can be done, but in fact exists within a Rogerian framework. For the purpose of this discussion, we are not talking about medical research, basic or clinical; nor are we making any comment regarding appropriateness or choice of medical therapies, including standard or unorthodox approaches. Standards of clinical practice do exist and are outlined elsewhere, and have little or no bearing on the *art* of practicing medicine. The assumption is tacitly made that the physician always acts in accordance with Hippocrates' classic charge of first doing no harm. It is to the manner in which medical practice is conducted that I would like to turn my attention. Simply put, it is the prospect of practicing from a unitary perspective. Any time a physician works with a patient, be it a brief encounter or long-term care, it can be viewed as a process. This process involves mutual appreciation and expectations, patient teaching, power enhancement, and, in Rogerian terms, commitment to the integral mutual process of patterning the human environmental field for the betterment of everyone. As defined above, these processes are mutually inclusive and to a large extent contemporaneous; the order in which they are discussed in no way implies that one necessarily occurs before another, or that where one ends the next begins. Rather, they are integral and to a large extent are all occurring simultaneously.

In the beginning, neither doctor nor patient knows if they will continue working with each other in the process of healthcare. Mutual appreciation and expectations are more important and complex than they may first appear. Patterns that characterize patients' views of who a doctor is and what he or she does emerge from the mutual processing of human environmental fields in the relative past and relative present. Historical and psychological antecedents, encompassing early cultures and traditions of healing, not routinely acknowledged in the doctor/patient milieu, are significant.

In most early cultures, the healer—shaman, and physician—traditionally occupied positions of some respect in their various societies, due to a combination of factors. First, they performed a service that was perceived as valuable, if not necessary for the society. Second, they were possessed of certain skills, or gifts, or training, which the other members of the society did not have; whether this was due to the vertical transmission of a presumed ability, such as was seen in the patrilineal inheritance patterns of primitive tribal shamans, or to the accumulation of skill and knowledge in academies of learning, as was the case in Greek and Roman civilizations, mattered little. The doctor was different, and this difference set him (and it was almost always a "him") apart. Third, and at least as important as the first two, there was an element of trust. The members of the society truly believed that the healer had the ability to heal. Here was perhaps the crux of the issue, for the belief that one is going to get well is critically important to the process of getting well. And last, but equally important, was the fact that people believed not only that the doctor could help, but also that he wanted to help; he was genuinely concerned. Being a doctor has, over the years, never been about only what you know and can do, but also about what the patient believes you know and can do, and about the manner in which you do it.

This was not the only view of doctors throughout history, of course, and the counterbalancing view is a sobering one. Medieval surgeons were glorified members of the barbers' guild, and that physicians, while generally held in some esteem because of their role, were often objects of popular derision, as witness their foppish and narcissistic portrayals in literature throughout the ages. During epidemics such as the Black Death, physicians were seen as impotent, and the more prudent of them, undoubtedly aware that they could do nothing for their patients, discarded their long-beaked masks filled with burning incense (to prevent spread of the plague), and fled the large cities for the more rural countryside.

The message is clear: Patients may believe they need us but they don't have to love us. They don't want to be lorded over, and they reserve the right to gleefully puncture our balloons of self-importance. They desperately want to put their trust in someone whom they feel knows more than they do and can help them, but they demand that the nature of that trust be honored on a human level. And as physicians, we owe them that.

Physicians also owe them the right to be viewed and appreciated as unitary human beings, recognizing that they have the capacity to knowingly participate in change (Barrett, 1990b). Rogers (1970) states that "nursing exists to serve people" (p. 112). Similarly, the scientific art of medical practice exists to serve people. While practicing from a Rogerian view, the physician collaborates and participates with the patient in their healing process, "facilitating the expression of a person's greatest potential" (Phillips, 1990, p. 17), rather than acting upon it. The physician must also respect and appreciate the uniqueness of each person who comes to them for healthcare.

All of this must be taken into account when considering the complex nature of the "doctor-patient relationship." Most patients coming to a doctor's office are looking for someone with knowledge and skill and with whom they can feel comfortable. They don't have to think we are infallible (good thing, since none of us are), but they do have to trust us. Living up to these expectations can be difficult.

PATTERNING THE HUMAN ENVIRONMENTAL FIELD

The office should be patterned to address the issue of "familiarity" in the sense that the decor is pleasant and tranquil, rather than portraying a cold, sterile atmosphere. Fresh flowers, current magazines, comfortable furniture, and soft music facilitate a sense of calmness. The office staff should be friendly, but not overly familiar, such as taking the liberty of addressing patients by their first names unless patients have made it clear that is what they want.

Patterning the environment also involves communicating a sense of friendly professionalism, but with a certain degree of reserve to promote confidence in the physician as a healer. Educational materials, the requisite diplomas on the walls, and the books on the shelves assist in patterning the surroundings to manifest a healing environment.

When I see a patient for the first time, I make it a point to go into the waiting room where I introduce myself with a handshake and bring them back into my office. Whether the patient is seeing me for a checkup or a highly specialized second opinion, I want the patient to identify me first as a human being and then as a doctor. Observing this simple social convention can be quite disarming. Unfortunately, many patients come to the office hoping to be helped but also expecting to be condescended to. I always wear a tie in the office; I may not wear my white coat, or I may loosen my tie a bit and open my collar, but I try to convey the idea that I have dressed for the occasion of the patient's visit. When we are in my office, I will often comment briefly, before we get to the medical issues, about some piece of information on the patient's registration sheet, such as asking about the person who may have referred them to me ("How is Arthur Jones? I haven't seen him in a while."), or about their listed occupation ("What exactly is a systems manager?"); the answers are never time-consuming, but the fact that I ask the question reassures the patient that I am interested in them as a person, not just a disease. While it is true that in most cases patients come to me for help with a specific condition, it is crucial that they know that the help is being proferred to a person by a person.

Pattern appraisal of the patient involves picking up subtle cues from what someone says or how they say it, how they sit in the chair, or which questions they answer obliquely, to formulate an overall gestalt of what they are like as a person. The pattern appraisal begins in the waiting room, upon first meeting, and proceeds through the entire history-taking and physical examination, to the final conference and throughout the length of the relationship. It is the process of gathering information about a patient—not about their disease, for they will be more than forthcoming about that, but about the person—so as to be in the position to address their needs, fears, hopes, and the like. This is a critical step, for without it there is no way to even contemplate the next step, that of engaging in mutual process with the patient for the purpose of healing, which is what the entire physician-patient process is supposed to be about. Although neither I nor most other physicians would ever dream of formulating it in these terms, it is the equivalent of Rogers' identification of energy field patterns.

We have all noted at one time or another that there are certain people who brighten up a room simply by being there, and there are others who seem to bring their own cloud with them to dampen any social gathering. These are the extreme examples of a basic phenomenon: Everyone has his or her unique energy field, whose pattern manifestations can be identified by others. In the case of the life of the party, the pattern manifestation is so strong as to be apparent to everyone; in most people, the manifestations are far more subtle. Nonetheless, those who would heal must train themselves to recognize pattern characteristics and to use them to create a unique and distinctive picture of the individual to be healed.

I observe the way the patient responds to my initial greeting, the purposefulness of the handshake, and the way he or she walks into the office. It is easy to distinguish the corporate executive in for a checkup with her determined stride from the terrified young man who has noticed some blood in his stool. An elderly woman who is immaculately dressed and walks slowly but with great grace is clearly a proud person who will always lend—and need—a dignified air to the encounter. In the initial interview, I always begin by saying "The floor is yours," or something on that order, to allow the patient to tell the story as he or she sees it. The way the history is presented, and especially any inconsistencies in that history or inappropriate emphasis on seemingly minor complaints, is often a very good clue to the reason for the visit. To miss these pattern manifestations is to miss what the patient is really there for.

For example, a middle-aged woman was in to see me recently for a complaint of rectal bleeding. She had been told of hemorrhoids years ago, and advised to do nothing for them as they were small. She had been colonoscoped three years before, and nothing was found, save for the hemorrhoids. The character or amount of the bleeding had not changed in the past ten years, and she had no other symptoms. She was not at increased risk for malignancy by virtue of family history or any other parameter, and the description of the bleeding was that of classic hemorrhoidal disease. She felt perfectly well. She described the bleeding symptoms in detail, and only on further questioning did she admit that those symptoms were not appreciably different from anything she had ever had before. It wasn't clear to me why she had suddenly come in for a consultation, until I asked her on a hunch if any close friend or relative had recently been diagnosed with any disease of the colon. She hesitated momentarily, then became tearful and admitted that her best friend since childhood had recently died of colon cancer. The loss was fresh, and it had transformed a whole set of symptoms with which she had been quite comfortable for years into harbingers of doom. Addressing the likelihood of having colon cancer with a negative colonoscopy three years ago based on polyp doubling times was not going to be fruitful, nor would dismissing the symptoms as hemorrhoidal. Once it was clear what her underlying fear was, it was easy enough to reassure her that the likelihood of this being due to cancer was very low, that the loss of her friend was figuring prominently in the causation of her anxiety, and that a simple sigmoidoscopy, for which she actually would be due soon anyway, would answer the question. She had the procedure, it was normal, and she remains well.

In this case, as in any number of others, the appraisal of the patient would have been incomplete if only the history and physical exam were taken at face value. The underlying disease was a temporary but incapacitating anxiety, which had the power to transform minor (but real) symptoms into clear-cut (to the patient) indicators of fatal disease. The physician's job is to heal; if the disease is anxiety, the anxiety must be addressed, not to the exclusion of the physical symptoms but as integral with them. Reassuring the patient that his or her symptoms are not fatal is not enough. We must recognize and validate the anxiety as being very real to that patient at that moment, respecting it and handling it as an independent entity, and recognizing that there are occasions where anxiety has saved lives.

Sometimes a patient will be accompanied to the office by a family member or close friend. The significance of the patient-other dyad should be noted, since it may indicate that the patient considers himself or herself, not only in life but also and specifically in the context of the illness, not as an individual but as a part of a unit. In Rogerian terms, this unit would be viewed as an energy field. While my first responsibility is to the patient alone, and the patient's privacy is always respected, if I ignore the significant other I do so at my own risk. Sometimes the other person is there only for moral support, sometimes because he or she is intimately involved in healthcare decisions; differentiating these aspects is usually easily done by observing the nature of the mutual process. If it is a close family member who is involved, they are often going to expect to be included in discussions and decisions, and if this is amenable to the patient, I make it a point to do so. In close family units, patients have needs and family members have needs, and both sets of needs must be addressed in treating the patient.

An example will illustrate this phenomenon. During my first year of practice, I was asked to see a woman in her late seventies because of dysphagia. She had been worked up in Florida and told of a benign esophageal stricture, and referred to another physician for dilatation. Her son brought her to New York for a second opinion, and I saw her with her x-rays and endoscopy reports. Before I actually saw her, I had two conversations with the son by phone, and he accompanied her to the office. He was very concerned about her; he was an only child, and the father had died when he was very young, leaving the mother and son as each other's only family member for years. The son was a very successful corporate executive who made it clear that he would spare no expense in his mother's care; his fiancee was a nurse who was willing to provide nursing input at home if needed. The patient herself was continually expressing her gratitude to her son throughout the consultation. It was a close and very powerful relationship.

My review of the x-rays raised a strong suspicion of esophageal carcinoma, and the patient underwent rigid esophagoscopy, which on deep biopsy confirmed the presence of malignancy. When I gave the son the report, his first concern was that his mother not be told yet, since she was agreeable to surgery if needed. He felt strongly that if she knew she had cancer she would definitely die. We agreed that she would be told only that the biopsy indicated that dilatation would be useless, and surgery was needed, to which she readily agreed. At the time of surgery, a large carcinoma was found with local extension into the mediastinum and metastatic deposits throughout the abdomen; a Celestin prothesis was placed and the patient was closed. Again the son prevailed upon me that the diagnosis not be given; he insisted that he knew his mother better than anyone, and that being given the diagnosis of cancer would kill her. As a physician, I feel strongly that patients have the right to know, and I have the duty to inform them of their diagnoses, but in the case of this 79-year-old woman, who had already said that she would refuse chemotherapy or radiation even if she needed it, I agreed to postpone giving her the news, at least until her postoperative healing was complete. The prosthesis enabled her to eat, and she recovered a significant amount of strength. Her son arranged care for her, and she continued to improve and gain weight. She moved to a nursing home, where she remained for eight years. A CAT scan done seven years after her surgery showed only thickening of the distal esophagus; no locally infiltrating or distantly metastatic disease could be seen.

Cases like this are not unheard-of, but I do believe that respecting the son's wishes not to inform his mother of her diagnosis added years to her life. And I do believe that had she known the diagnosis, she would have been dead in the expected six months. I also believe, based on what I knew of this family, that acting in accordance with his wishes was the same as acting in accordance with her wishes, and the outcome was the best it could have been under the circumstances.

This case not only illustrates the importance of seeing the patient as a unitary human being, but also demonstrates the integrality of the human environmental energy field. Although all of what we have discussed—evaluating the family structure, picking up cues from patient behavior in the office, "getting the vibes," if you will—may seem time-consuming, most of it is actually done almost reflexively and is ongoing during the history and examination, not apart from it. Appraising the patient—identifying the energy field patterning—is essential for the next step to occur.

PARTICIPATING IN THE MUTUAL PROCESSING OF HUMAN ENVIRONMENTAL ENERGY FIELDS

How one participates in the mutual process of human environmental energy fields is the heart of the matter; everything else is a prelude. Based on the pattern appraisal, one proceeds with deliberative mutual patterning (Barrett, 1990a). This is nothing more than taking what you know of the patient, in the context of your relationship with the patient, and letting yourself act in a natural way with the desire of doing the right thing for him. It involves taking the identified need of a fatigued patient (for example, fear of leukemia because a friend had leukemia and her symptoms started off with fatigue), using your skills at history-taking and physical examination to reassure the patient (nothing in the history suggests a myeloproliferative disorder, and the examination is entirely normal), using the established trust to put credence behind your reassurance (you've seen patients with leukemia, and based on that experience, you think this diagnosis is unlikely), and using the tools you have at your disposal to evaluate the situation and arrive at the ultimate conclusion (a blood count will be checked, and if normal, will rule out leukemia). There is nothing terribly sophisticated about this approach, and it is something most of us do daily. But it is why patients feel better, and that is after all what our job is about.

Some physicians feel that once they have made a diagnosis and gotten that patient to the appropriate specialist, their role is over; in most cases, that is just not true. If your intent is to be the patient's doctor, making the diagnosis is only the beginning of your involvement. As physicians, we often forget that for the patient, experiencing a serious illness is a journey into an uncharted sea, and being cared for by a multiplicity of specialists is akin to being cut adrift in that sea, having to navigate one's own way from island to island. Most patients depend on their doctor to guide them, to be the central repository of accumulated data, and to be the source of ongoing support in the healing process. When a patient with pancreatic cancer asks me if her oncologist has kept me informed about the latest change in her chemotherapy, my initial thought is, "Why would he? What input could—or should—I have into a specialized area I know nothing about?" But to take her question at face value is to miss the point. She trusts her oncologist, but she needs to know that somewhere in the vast pool of modern medicine into which she has been unceremoniously dumped, there is one physician who is at her side through the whole process. Whether I know the dose of 5-FU she is receiving, or even the name of the experimental agent in her IV bottle, is immaterial; what is happening to her is being cleared through her physician-advocate, and that helps to make it all right.

There are other ways for the mutual process to occur in caring for patients. Some of these are so subtle as to be manifest not in words, but in behavioral cues that we transmit to patients, and what they do is reinforce to the patient that there is another human being—a little less than kin, and more than kind—at their side through it all. Extensive studies have been done on the role of touch, not only such formalized concepts as

Therapeutic Touch, but simply the role of physical touch in psychological and social bonding (Heidt, 1981; Keller & Bzdek, 1986; Krieger, 1988; Moyers, 1995, pp. 230, 338, 356). In the physician-patient energy field process, physical touch is the bridge that helps communicate the depth of healing desire on the part of the healer. Whether in the handshake upon entering the exam room, or by sitting on the patient's hospital bed and resting a hand on his shoulder during a discussion, the touch of the doctor's hand communicates not only empathy but also the power to heal; witness the time-honored expression for the ultimate in healing, "laying on of the hands."

TEACHING PATIENTS

Teaching patients is one area in which physicians have been regrettably lax. Perhaps because of the traditional authoritarian/paternalistic model of the "doctor-patient relationship," physicians have expected patients to follow directions and have not laid much emphasis to explanation. There is also the fact that most patients simply wanted to get better, without long discourses on disease mechanism; that may still be true today. Last, there is the time factor; as physicians have gotten busier, and time has come to be at a premium, there is barely enough time to treat, let alone explain. The advent of managed care will do nothing to improve this situation; it will render it more impossible than ever. So there would seem to be little justification for including teaching in the physician's role.

Or is there? The traditional authoritarian model is fast disappearing. Patients are becoming more involved in their care, and more proactive about it. Over and over we hear patients ask, what can I do about this? What can I do to help myself? Physicians can hardly expect blind obedience from patients, nor should they. The patient is the one with the disease, and in the evolving paradigm of healthcare, must accept some responsibility for his or her own well-being. As a physician, I may not be able to force a patient to stop smoking. I can—and do—tell the patient all the dangers of smoking, enumerating the conditions that it can cause and the consequences thereof. I then tell them that I'm available to try to help them to stop, if they want to stop; that I can't make them stop if they don't want to; and end by appealing to their intelligence to try to avoid the consequences of continued smoking. If they continue to smoke, that becomes their choice. Similarly, a patient with chronic ulcerative colitis will be encouraged to ask me questions about pathophysiology and pharmacotherapy, and I'll explain as much as they want to hear (and as much as I know). It is only with some understanding of their disease process that they can begin to take care of themselves—and most importantly, feel that they have some control over what is happening to them. With chronic disease, much of it is about control.

Barrett (1990) defines power as the capacity to participate knowingly in change. Patients experience illness in many ways, and one of the most important of these is as a loss of power. They don't feel well and so may not be able to do all the things they would like (loss of power of daily routine); there is some disruption in physical functioning (loss of power over their body); they have been forced to seek help from and put themselves in the hands of—read, "in the power of"—some other individual (loss of independence). Losing sense of power is a frightening experience. One of the things that physicians can do is to give patients back some sense of power by making what is happening to them less foreign, and that is best accomplished by education. Again, no one (least of all me, as a practicing physician for whom time management is hardly a forte) is suggesting that we try to teach patients to become their own doctors, exquisitely updated on and conversant with the finest details of disease mechanisms and management. In dealing with patients, however, a little education often goes a long way, especially if what is presented is germane to their daily functioning and not too abstruse. The patient with ulcerative colitis needs to know about dietary manipulations, and that the disease is an "autoimmune" reaction to the lining of the bowel, which we treat with certain anti-inflammatory medications that have been shown to bring patients into remission and, if taken continuously, to maintain remission. All of this information helps them on a day-to-day basis, and gives a rationale for the continued administration of medication even after the symptoms have improved. It is a rare patient who needs to know, or could conceivably do anything with, the mechanism of interleukin-2 release from inflammatory cells as a central part of the disease pathogenesis. When the patient with colitis asks me if he can stop his Azulfidine, since he has had no flare up in the last three years, how can I forbid it? I tell him that there is a good chance that the reason he has had no flare up is because of the drug, and that we know that when patients stop Azulfidine there is a good chance of disease reactivation. Do they all reactivate? No. Can I promise him that if he stops the drug his disease will flare up? No, no more than I can promise him that if he continues it he will never have another attack. What I can do is to give him the data he needs to enter into a decision-making process, give him my considered opinion (sometimes a strong opinion, sometimes less so), and help him to make the decision. By doing so, I am allowing him to participate in his own health-care management, giving him back some power in his life, and allowing for knowing participation in change—enhancing his power.

Enhancement of power springs from the idea that all people have within themselves some capacity for self-healing, and that we as physicians and nurses act to a degree as facilitators for that self-healing. This also represents a deviation from the authoritarian model of the "doctor-patient relationship," for it posits a collaborative effort directed at facilitating a potential source of power to heal from within the patient. Power enhancement emerges from the mutual process of human/environmental energy fields. It establishes a sense of control within realistic parameters. Power enhancement is the antithesis of abject helplessness and must be considered as being integral with the therapeutic process.

Power enhancement is more than simply giving information; it involves encouraging the patient to use information to make decisions, in the relative present or the relative future, and to act on those decisions as he or she sees fit. Barrett (1990b) defines power enhancement as "clients using their capacity to participate knowingly in change to actualize certain potentials" (p. 34). Power enhancement involves facilitating awareness, choices, freedom to act intentionally, and involvement in creating change (Barrett, 1990). Sometimes, enhancing power in a patient who has been passive in his or her healthcare can be gratifying for that patient.

I have taken care of Mrs. X for over ten years. She is a gracious, distinguished, well-dressed, and articulate widow in her early eighties who has mild hypertension and occasional episodes of tachycardia, which are both controlled with a calcium-channel blocker. An elevated cholesterol is controlled by diet. Over the years, we have found that although her hypertension is controlled, she gets anxious visiting the office and occasionally has higher readings there (so-called "white coat effect"), which are normalized if she engages in a simple mental exercise for a minute before I take her pressure (she closes her eyes, breathes deeply, and goes through the steps of making a cheesecake in her kitchen in the country). The fact that I allow her to do this has cemented our relationship, although it would be nice to think that bringing her through a particularly bad episode of diverticulitis may also have had something to do with this. In any event, she follows her diet strictly, although the salt "issue" has always upset her. Every physician she has ever seen has proscribed salt completely; she has seen more dietitians for sodium-restricted menus than anyone else I know. We were all taught in medical school that salt restriction is one of the earliest therapeutic maneuvers for hypertension, but Mrs. X has had it drummed into her that the stuff was absolute poison. In fact, her hypertension is mild and easily controlled, and she has never been anywhere near congestive heart failure. One day, we were talking in my office after her examination. I mentioned that I would be checking her cholesterol.

"I've been very good with my diet," she said, "although it kills me." I looked at her; she had never complained before about the diet. "What kills you?"

"I'm dying for a pastrami sandwich from the Second Avenue Deli." "When was the last time you had one?" I asked. She looked at me mournfully. "It's been years," she sighed. "I was always told not to, because of the salt and the fat."

This seemed unfair to me. Mrs. X's hypertension was hardly so severe that one pastrami sandwich was going to hurt her, and the fat in the sandwich was not going to push her cholesterol permanently into the danger zone. She was not lamenting the absence of pastrami from her daily diet; she had not tasted it in years.

I wrote out her prescriptions and handed them to her across the desk. Then I wrote out another prescription, on my blank, and handed it to her as well. It said:

PASTRAMI SANDWICH
#1
SIG: AS DIRECTED, PRUDENTLY

"You're a smart woman," I said, "and you know all about low-salt and low-cholesterol diets. Now I'm telling you that you can have the occasional pastrami sandwich when you want one. You can't make a habit of it, but if you have one occasionally, I can promise you you're not going to get into any trouble. If you do it too often, you'll start to retain water. But if you do it infrequently, you don't have to worry, and you can consider it doctor's orders."

She had a huge smile on her face as she carefully folded the prescription and put it in her purse. She still carries it there to this day, and it has given her a real sense of power and participation in her own care. When several years later her children threw her an eightieth birthday party at an elegant Manhattan restaurant, I was invited and was honored to hear myself thanked from the dais for being "the doctor who had faith in me and wrote me a prescription for my beloved pastrami sandwich." I don't know if she ever actually had the sandwich, but she knows that she can if she wants to, within limits that she and I have set up. So far, I haven't been called for any diuretics. This example illustrates that healing often involves the physician having faith in the patient, not just the patient having faith in the physician. It is a deliberate mutual patterning that promotes well-being. As Rogers noted, the notion of patient "compliance" is antithetical to practice reflecting the Science of Unitary Human Beings.

COMMITMENT TO THE INTEGRALITY
OF MUTUAL PROCESS

Committing to the integrality of continuous mutual process of human environmental energy fields involves knowing oneself and one's patient well enough to know when one or another aspect of the relationship should temporarily take precedence, always having as its prime mover the commitment to the patient as an integral and irreducible human being. It is the Hippocratic Oath, the fact that physician and patient have entered into a holy trust, and the fact that we recognize the necessary plasticity of that relationship within those confines. At its most basic, it states that I am open to healing you and will use every resource I can muster to do that; that you are open to being healed, and will use every resource at your disposal to help; and that we do this in an environment of ongoing respect and trust. It is in some ways the most amorphous aspect, but in many ways the most fundamental, for physicians, as well as any healthcare professional whose intent is to heal.

THE PLACE OF ROGERIAN PRACTICE IN
THE MANAGED CARE ENVIRONMENT

American medicine is undergoing a major change in the way it operates, due mainly to the advent of managed care. It would seem upon first glance that changes in medicine are not only inconsistent with, but also antithetical to, many of the concepts of Rogerian science. The need to enter into awareness of the mutual process with a patient, the appraisal of energy field patterns and the reconstitution of wholeness and well-being which underlie the Science of Unitary Human Beings; how do these possibly fit into a system in which cost-effectiveness is the bottom line, in which a premium is placed on seeing the most patients in the least time (for this concept underlies the directives given to physician employees of some HMOs)? In a system in which paperwork is spiraling and in which patients are moved in and out of physician panels as often as their employers change insurance carriers, where is the time for or the possibility of establishing the kind of interpersonal bond which the doctor-patient relationship presupposes? What is the CPT code for mutual process appraisal?

It is not going to be easy, but it can be done. One way to do it is to sensitize physicians to the nature of "doctor-patient relationships," so that they become more adept at recognizing and implementing the key aspects early on. The idea that physicians can "wing it" in this regard, or that a bad bedside manner can be excusable, is on its way to becoming an anachronism. An effort needs to be made to educate physicians at the medical school or immediate post-graduate level in aspects of clinical practice mechanics, an area that exists minimally, if at all in most curricula today. When these basic principles are internalized, they become second nature and practicing Rogerian medicine becomes no more time-intensive than medical practice ever was.

Another change occurring is the concept of physician extenders, practitioners who function in physician-adjunctive (or in some cases physician-equivalent) roles in a physician-based practice, such as nurse practitioners and physician assistants. Doctors in practice are currently being placed under pressure to see more and more patients in less and less time. The impetus for this is not only maintaining their current levels of income, but also being cost- and time-efficient so as to remain competitive for managed care contracts, without which there is a very bleak economic prospect. Under this kind of pressure, attention to Rogerian mutual processes with patients will often be difficult. The presence of a nurse practitioner, who cannot only handle medical problems but may also have more time to devote to the scientific art of nursing practice, will be a boon to the practice and a source of satisfaction to the patient.

One of the major changes in medicine is the shift from treatment to prevention of disease, and the maintenance of health. This is a paradigm shift that medical schools are only beginning to address, but that patients and insurers are demanding. The important contributions of other healthcare professionals and the unique sciences on which their practices are based will become increasingly evident in the new healing paradigm. Alternative as well as conventional therapies will continue to expand and patients will be increasingly involved in participating in their care. One problem with this turn of events—a problem primarily for physicians, since we were trained in a different mode—is that prevention and healing (with all the latter term implies) is far more laborious, more time-consuming, than simply fixing a problem. It takes more time to counsel a patient about smoking, to explore with him why he smokes, or why he has no desire to quit, to see what, if any ramifications his home life, or his job, or even his diet and nutritional status, have, than it does to write a prescription for an antibiotic each time he develops bronchitis, or to refer him to the pulmonologist when he develops emphysema, or to the oncologist when he develops lung cancer.

In my practice, which is probably a typically busy Manhattan one, I rarely have the time to do much counseling in the office; seeing sick people, doing diagnostic workups, answering calls from patients, making hospital rounds, and teaching make for a fairly full schedule. How would a nurse collaborate in this practice? By concentrating on health maintenance, by doing patient education, by using specific nursing modalities such as Therapeutic Touch as complementary treatment within the framework of a physician-nurse collaborative practice, with the overall goal being the delivery of highest quality healthcare not only to the seriously ill, but to everyone. Not only is the physician then able to better direct attention to where it is needed (a patient with an illness in the physician's area of greatest expertise, for example; or to teaching, writing, research, or other academic pursuits), but that physician is also able to devote more time in his or her practice to talking to the patients, to finding out what is bothering them, to working with that information and his or her own skills toward promoting well-being—in short, to healing them. Stress management, Therapeutic Touch, imagery techniques, field pattern appraisal, and deliberate mutual patterning—all of these will be used as important adjuncts to the practice of medicine. And there is simply not enough time or training for physicians to do it all.

CONCLUSION

The changes in healthcare in the last ten years have provided new opportunities to examine and evaluate the nature of many aspects of that healthcare. The mutual process of doctors and patients has recently been one aspect written about extensively (Crawshaw et al, 1995; Emanuel & Dubler, 1995; Glass, 1996; Siegler, 1993). Although no one has the answer (and no one knows what further changes or retrenchments healthcare will undergo in the coming years, and how this will impact healthcare providers), we as physicians must, to paraphrase John Balint and Wayne Shelton (Balint & Shelton, 1996), regain the initiative and forge a new model of that mutual process. The model proposed herein is a working one that a great number of physicians already employ at some level, and that is usually employed without even thinking about it. It can however be defined and implemented in a systematic, scientific, and teachable way, which happens to be highly consistent with many of the principles set down by Martha Rogers in her creation of the science for nursing practice. Rogerian science has much to teach physicians and nurses about healthcare and healing. This is fortunate, for we all have much to learn.

REFERENCES

Balint, J., & Shelton, W. (1996). Regaining the initiative: Forging a new model of the patient-physician relationship. *Journal of the American Medical Association, 275,* 887–891.

Barrett, E. A. M. (1990a). Health patterning with clients in a private practice environment. In E. A. M. Barrett (Ed.), *Visions of Rogers' science-based nursing* (pp. 110–115). New York: NLN Press.

Barrett, E. A. M. (1990b). Rogers' science-based nursing practice. In E. A. M. Barrett (Ed.), *Visions of Rogers' science-based nursing* (pp. 31–44). New York: NLN Press.

Crawshaw, R., Rogers, D., & Pellegrino, E. (1995). Patient-physician covenant. *Journal of the American Medical Association, 273,* 1553.

Emanuel, E., & Dubler, N. (1995). Preserving the physician-patient relationship in the era of managed care. *Journal of the American Medical Association, 273,* 323–329.

Glass, R. (1996). The patient-physician relationship. *Journal of the American Medical Association, 275(2),* 147–148.

Heidt, P. (1981). Effect of therapeutic touch on the anxiety level in hospitalized patients. *Nursing Research, 30,* 32–37.

Keller, E., & Bzdek, V. M. (1986). Effects of therapeutic touch on tension headache pain. *Nursing Research, 35(2),* 101–106.

Krieger, D. (1988). *Therapeutic touch: Two decades of research, teaching, and clinical practice.* Paper presented at the twentieth anniversary of Council Grove Conferences on Voluntary Controls Program for the Menninger Foundation, Topeka, KS.

Moyers, B. (1995). *Healing and the mind.* New York: Doubleday.

Phillips, J. R. (1990). Changing human potentials and future visions of nursing: A human field image perspective. In E. A. M. Barrett (Ed.), *Visions of Rogers' science-based nursing* (pp. 13–25). New York: NLN Press.

Rogers, M. E. (1970). *Introduction to the theoretical basis of nursing.* Philadelphia: Davis.

Rogers, M. E. (1994). Nursing science evolves. In M. Madrid & E. A. M. Barrett (Eds.), *Rogers' scientific art of nursing practice* (pp. 3–9). New York: NLN Press.

Siegler, M. (1993). Falling off the pedestal: What is happening to the traditional doctor-patient relationships? *Mayo Clinic Procedure, 68,* 461–467.

Appendix

GLOSSARY

Energy Field: The fundamental unit of the living and the nonliving. Field is a unifying concept. Energy signifies the dynamic nature of the field. A field is in continuous motion and is infinite.

Pattern: The distinguished characteristics of an energy field perceived as a single wave.

Pandimensional: A nonlinear domain without spatial or temporal attributes.

Unitary Human Being: An irreducible, indivisible, pandimensional energy field identified by pattern and manifesting characteristics that are specific to the whole and which cannot be predicted from knowledge of the parts.

Environment: An irreducible, pandimensional energy field identified by pattern and integral with the human field.

Power: The capacity to participate knowingly in the nature of change characterizing the continuous patterning of the human and environmental fields as manifest by awareness, choices, freedom to act intentionally, and involvement in creating change. (Barrett, 1990, p. 108)

PRINCIPLES OF HOMEODYNAMICS

Resonancy: Continuous change from lower to higher frequency wave patterns in human and environmental fields.

Helicy: Continuous, innovative, unpredictable, increasing diversity of human and environmental field patterns.

Integrality: Continuous mutual human field and environmental field process.

285

REFERENCES

Barrett, E. A. M. (1990). Health patterning with clients in a private practice environment. In E. A. M. Barrett (Ed.), *Visions of Rogers' science-based nursing* (pp. 105-115). New York: NLN Press.

Rogers, M. E. (1990). Nursing: Science of unitary, irreducible human beings: Update 1990. In E. A. M. Barrett (Ed.), *Visions of Rogers' science-based nursing* (pp. 5-11). New York: NLN Press.

MANIFESTATIONS OF FIELD PATTERNING IN UNITARY HUMAN BEINGS

The evolution of unitary human beings is a dynamic, irreducible, nonlinear process characterized by increasing diversity of energy field patterning. Manifestations of patterning emerge out of the human/environmental field mutual process and are continuously innovative. Pattern is an abstraction that reveals itself through its manifestations.

The nature of unitary field patterning is unpredictable and creative. Change is relative and increasingly diverse. Some manifestations of relative diversity in field patterning are noted below:

lesser diversity		greater diversity
longer rhythms	shorter rhythms	seems continuous
slower motion	faster motion	seems continuous
time experienced as slower	time experienced as faster	timelessness
pragmatic	imaginative	visionary
longer sleeping	longer waking	beyond waking

Rogers, M. E. (1990). Nursing: Science of unitary, irreducible human beings: Update 1990. In E. A. M. Barrett (Ed.), *Visions of Rogers' science-based nursing* (pp. 5-11). New York: NLN Press.

Index